ESSENTIAL SPORTS NUTRITION

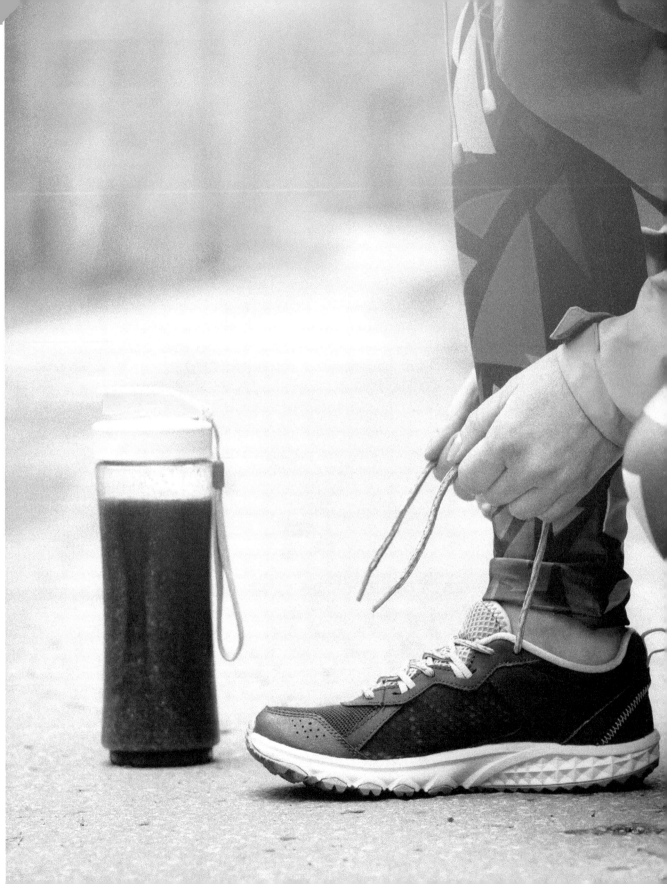

Essential Sports Nutrition

A GUIDE TO OPTIMAL PERFORMANCE
FOR EVERY ACTIVE PERSON

Marni Sumbal, MS, RD, CSSD, LD/N

ROCKRIDGE
PRESS

To my dad who taught me to always add life to my years and never give up on my dreams.

Cover photography © Shutterstock/baibaz (front cover, granola); Shutterstock/topseller (front cover, ribbon); Shutterstock/ostill (back cover)
Interior photography © Shutterstock/LMproduction (page ii); Shutterstock/Foxys Forest Manufacture (page vii)
Author photo © Joey Mock

Cover Design: William Mack
Interior Design: Meg Woodcheke
Editor: Vanessa Ta
Production Editor: Erum Khan

ISBN: Print 978-1-64152-169-7 | eBook 978-1-64152-170-3

R2

CONTENTS

Preface vi

Introduction vii

PART ONE **How What We Consume Affects Our Bodies** 1

1   Nutrition Sources 3

2   Components of an Optimal Diet 29

PART TWO **Nutrient Timing for Better Results** 50

3   Fueling Before Exercise 52

4   Fueling During and After Exercise 61

5   Fueling on Rest Days 74

6   Supplements and Performance Enhancers 81

PART THREE **Optimal Performance for Every Athlete** 89

7   Factors Affecting Nutrition Needs 90

8   Considerations for Men and Women 94

9   Considerations for Children and Student Athletes 100

10 Sport-Specific Nutrition Needs 106

11 Nutrition for Weight Loss, Weight Gain, and Weight Maintenance 115

12 Nutrition for Recovery and Immune Function 120

13 Body and Brain 130

PART FOUR **Recipes for Success** 134

14 Recipes for Before Exercise or Competition 135

15 Recipes for During and After Exercise 143

16 Recipes for Rest Days 153

Glossary 162

Resources 168

References 169

Index 175

Recipe Index 181

PREFACE

As a board-certified sports dietitian, I've worked with countless individuals over the years who have sought nutrition assistance for fitness or sport improvement. I've consulted with athletes and exercise enthusiasts of all levels and backgrounds whose goals have included the desire to change their body composition, better their overall health, and improve their athletic performance. I've been asked so many nutrition questions about the best strategies that an athlete can pursue to reach athletic goals. How can I avoid stomach issues during workouts? Can I become a stronger athlete on a vegetarian diet? Do I need sports drinks if I'm not an elite athlete? How can I avoid dehydration? What should I eat to recover faster and reduce inflammation?

My answers to these and other nutrition questions are rooted in the last decade of my practice in exercise physiology and sports nutrition. But I also have personal experience. In addition to my career, I'm an endurance triathlete, having completed 13 Ironman-distance triathlons. These one-day, extreme endurance races ask a lot of my body. I know that if I don't properly fuel, hydrate, and nourish my body, I can't perform to my potential, and ultimately my health will suffer.

I've built my career on the belief that the best fitness routines and training strategies are only beneficial if your body is properly fueled and nourished. The best way to optimize performance without disrupting health is to rely on realistic, effective, and simple sports nutrition information. Only then can you help your body safely adapt to exercise. If you desire relevant, evidence-based sports nutrition advice and strategies that don't rely on extreme practices or restrictive measures, then this book is for you. In *Essential Sports Nutrition*, I unpack all of the nutrition information you'll need to make the most of your workout or sport so you can reach athletic excellence with a nutritionally rich style of eating.

INTRODUCTION

On a basic level, nutrition reduces your risk of disease and provides a source of energy so you can perform daily activities—but for the extremely active person, what and when you eat is crucial to helping you meet performance goals without creating health-related setbacks. Sports nutrition can be confusing, but it's essential to enhancing your body's adaptation to exercise. When you put science-based principles into practice, you'll find it much easier to perform to your potential.

Your athletic ability or performance involves more than the latest gear, strong muscles, and a great coach. Solid nutrition habits are the foundation for any fitness plan, whether you're training for competition or exercising for health. Supply your body with the right nutrients at the right times, and you'll be consistently rewarded with high energy, great health, and quick recovery. The right kind of diet also reduces your risk of sickness, injury, and burnout.

When you exercise, your energy demands increase. The foods you eat fuel your body with that energy. If your body doesn't receive the appropriate fuel, you'll perform well below your capabilities. As the duration or intensity of exercise increases, your body is challenged to keep up with energy demands. That's when fatigue occurs. Fall short on your fueling requirements and you can sabotage your physical health and your psychological well-being.

Sports performance and activity enjoyment depend on many different but intertwined components: body composition, strength, endurance, psychology, sleep. Yet many athletes are misled to believe that there's only one "right" way to eat. I often hear from my athletes that dairy is bad or that sugar is off-limits during competition season. Right now, the current sports nutrition trend is to restrict carbohydrate intake. I tell athletes that being mindful of what you eat is important, but adhering to only one set of sports nutrition principles is short-sighted. Applying a restrictive approach to sports nutrition often ignores long-term health and performance consequences—especially if the diet is seen as a "quick fix" to boost performance or change body composition. In this book, I take a more all-inclusive approach. I'll give you practical nutrition strategies to help you enhance sports performance, fitness, and long-lasting health. I hope you find this book easy to follow, with essential guidelines to apply to your active lifestyle.

There is no definitive standard prescription for sports nutrition. However, in this book I'll help you move closer to creating a personalized nutrition plan while gaining knowledge and appreciation for sports nutrition.

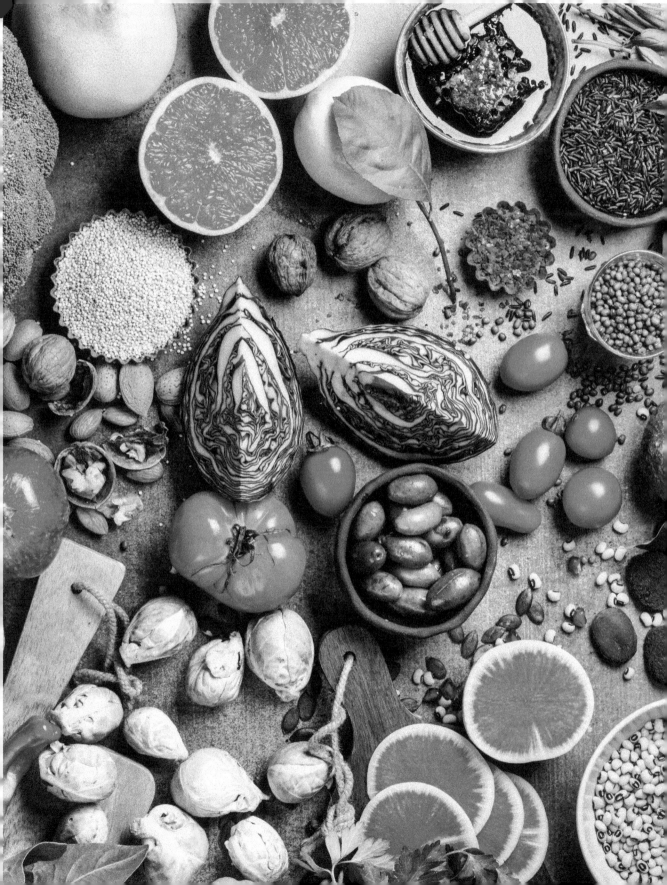

PART ONE

How What We Consume Affects Our Bodies

Food is your fuel. Eating should never cause anxiety, worry, or frustration. Unfortunately, that isn't always the case. We all come to the table with a unique food history that shouldn't be ignored when devising your personal nutrition plan. For example, you may value the importance of home-cooked meals, but your long work hours make it exhausting to meal prep. Perhaps you understand the principles of healthy eating but don't enjoy cooking. Maybe your family's budget is tight, so you often rely on less expensive, processed foods to stretch the dollar. And in our weight- and image-obsessed culture, trying to match your energy intake to your energy output may be tricky if you have a complicated relationship with food. In our fast-paced society, work, school, and other life commitments make it challenging to support the intense demands of physical activity. But for your body to remain in good health, your diet is key. You should strive for optimal nutrition in both quantity and quality. This means taking the time to learn about the nutrients that your body needs to function properly and having a practical game plan for how to turn that knowledge into action. ➤

For example:

- Water helps you maintain body temperature and remove waste, and it also lubricates your joints.

- Carbohydrates provide energy for your muscles, help maintain blood glucose levels, and fuel the central nervous system.

- Proteins are the building blocks of your muscles and aid with rapid recovery after a workout.

- Fat is an essential nutrient that provides energy while supporting body functions necessary for human health.

- Vitamins and minerals optimize immune system health and provide the spark for metabolic reactions that turn food into energy during exercise.

No single food can boost your health or performance. Rather, it's the synergy of all the foods in your diet that affects bodily functions during exercise.

1
CHAPTER

Nutrition Sources

The human body is amazing. At rest, it's under minimal stress. Little work is required to sleep, work, or stare at your smartphone. During exercise, however, your body's systems are put into high gear as they experience great physiological stress. These include hormonal, neurotransmitter, metabolic, and enzymatic reactions. To optimize these processes, you must regularly provide your body with high-quality sources of energy and nutrients from the food you eat.

Unfortunately, many athletes neglect proper eating until a setback occurs. I'm here to say that it's never too late to appreciate the power of food. By keeping track of your fuel, nutrient, and hydration needs, you can protect your health, delay fatigue, and consistently improve your fitness.

In this chapter, you will learn the importance of dietary carbohydrates, protein, fat, and water, and about their impact on the health and function in the body during exercise. It's imperative to consider the combination of foods in your diet instead of viewing your diet in single-food components. Remember, you're made up of what you consume, and what you consume affects your health and performance.

Fluids and Electrolytes

Although water has no caloric value, it's the most essential nutrient required by your body on a daily basis. Humans are made of water. It's part of your blood, brain, heart, lungs, and bones. At birth, your total body weight is about 75 percent water. When you are an adult, that amount decreases to 50 to 65 percent. For example, an adult who weighs 150 pounds carries about 40 liters (88 pounds) of fluid inside the body! This number changes inversely with fat mass, meaning more fat equals less water. Water plays many important roles in your body, and you simply can't survive without it.

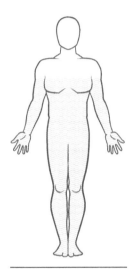

- Water transports glucose, oxygen, and fatty acids through your blood to working muscles.
- Water eliminates metabolic waste products such as carbon dioxide and lactic acid in the form of urine.
- Water absorbs heat from your muscles during exercise and dissipates it through sweat via the skin, ultimately regulating body temperature.
- Water helps digest food through saliva and gastric secretions.
- Water lubricates joints and cushions organs and tissues.
- Water nourishes the brain and spinal cord.
- Water is where all biochemical reactions occur.

Water plays many important roles in your body and makes up between 50-65 percent of your body weight.

Even though you're made of water, you still need to drink it, too. Every day you lose 2 to 3 liters of water from sweating, urinating, breathing, and bowel movements. Ensuring that you're adequately hydrated is essential to your health. Water isn't your only source of hydration, though. Foods such as cabbage, celery, grapes, melon, and zucchini can help as well.

The water inside your body contains **electrolytes**, which produce both positively and negatively charged ions. These ions conduct electrical activity and consist of sodium and chloride, magnesium, potassium, and calcium. The electrolytes must contain precise concentrations of ions in the blood, specifically sodium and potassium, in order to support fluid balance, muscle contractions, and neuron activity. Too many or too few can cause health issues. For example, cardiac issues can result from increased potassium in your bloodstream. Your kidneys are equipped to constantly adjust water levels and stave off an imbalance of electrolytes.

Five main electrolytes inside your body

ELECTROLYTE	ROLE IN THE BODY	MAIN FOOD SOURCES
Sodium and chloride	Maintain fluid balance and blood pressure, transmit nerve signals	Salt (40 percent sodium, 60 percent chloride) 1 tsp. salt = 2,300mg sodium
Potassium	Conducts nerve impulses and muscle contractions; crucial to heart function	Cooked winter squash, sweet potatoes, white potatoes, white beans, yogurt, milk, bananas
Calcium	Regulates heartbeat, assists in muscle contractions and nerve signals	Milk, yogurt, kefir, cheese, kale, watercress, bok choy, sardines
Magnesium	Maintains normal muscle and heart rhythm, conducts nerve impulses	Spinach, Swiss chard, whole grains, almonds, pumpkin seeds, dark chocolate, beans

To better understand the role of electrolytes in maintaining fluid balance, it's important to understand where fluid is found in the body.

Intracellular: The space within your cells makes up two-thirds of your total body fluid.

Extracellular: The space between your cells makes up one-third of your total body fluid.

Body cavity: The fluid here is known as transcellular fluid, such as cerebral spinal fluid and synovial, peritoneal, and pleural fluids, and it makes up only 3 percent of your total body fluid.

For the body to function normally, it must keep fluid levels from fluctuating too much in these areas. When an adjustment is needed, the body actively moves electrolytes in and out of cells. Because water moves freely between compartments, having electrolytes in the proper concentrations is important for maintaining fluid balance within the compartments. This balanced state is called homeostasis.

Extracellular fluid (ECF)

Interstitial fluid

Intracellular fluid (ICF)

Plasma (intravascular fluids)

Body Fluids and Fluid Compartments.

Fluid is found in the extracellular space within your body. Roughly 20 percent is in the vascular space, and 80 percent is in the interstitial space—that's the area between cells and blood vessels. Although these fluid compartments are classified as separate areas, the electrolytes and water in your body constantly flow between them. This ensures that the composition of each stays fairly constant.

The key to a properly functioning body is to ensure that your fluid intake closely matches your fluid loss on a day-to-day basis. You need to ingest water and electrolytes from food and drinks to keep plasma volume and **osmolality** at normal levels. Your thirst mechanism is a reliable way to help maintain fluid balance on a daily basis.

Your kidneys are ultimately responsible for the balance of fluids and solutes in your body. They get help from the **antidiuretic hormone (ADH)** and **aldosterone**. Total fluid volume in your body is typically maintained within 1 percent on a daily basis. But fluid balance can be thrown off by sweating, fluid intake, vomiting, and diarrhea.

By drinking an adequate amount of fluid during exercise, you can minimize **dehydration** and optimize the sweat response. Fluid also helps control core body temperature, aids in digestion, and reduces cardiovascular stress. Although dehydration may not always immediately impair performance, it will eventually reduce aerobic endurance, cognitive function, and anaerobic power.

Dehydration and Overhydration Symptoms to Keep in Mind

MILD DEHYDRATION

- Reduced performance
- Headache
- Fatigue
- Impaired cognition
- Less-elastic skin
- Sunken eyes
- Dry mouth
- Dizziness
- Loss of appetite
- Increased thirst

EXTREME DEHYDRATION

- Hypotension
- Tachycardia
- Weak pulse
- Cold hands/chills
- Reduced urination
- Shrunken brain
- Organ failure
- Death

OVERHYDRATION

- Nausea
- Vomiting
- Headache
- Puffy face, hands, and ankles
- Changes in mental state
- Muscle weakness, cramps, and spasms
- Seizures

A change in body weight, both pre- and post-exercise, is a practical way to assess hydration status. Significant weight loss, between 1 percent and 5 percent, can cause dehydration symptoms. Weight gain may represent overhydration. Hyponatremia is often associated with ultra-endurance athletes who drink too much plain water. Weight fluctuations are normal throughout the day—that's because bowel movements, food intake, inflammation, and glycogen depletion all affect your weight. **Glycogen** is the storage form of carbohydrates that's stored in the body for fuel. I talk more about this later on in the chapter.

Urine color also says a lot about your hydration status. When you are dehydrated, the kidneys filter waste to retain water, which causes urine to become darker and more concentrated. Certain supplements, foods, and medications, including B vitamins, rhubarb, and beet juice, may alter urine color. Some antibiotics and anti-inflammatory medications may also change the color. If your urine appears cloudy, it may be a medical ailment, such as a urinary tract infection or kidney stones. See your doctor for a diagnosis and proper treatment.

Urine color and hydration status

COLOR	HYDRATION STATUS
	Pale yellow to clear = well hydrated
	Light yellow = ideal hydration
	Moderate yellow = okay but rehydration needed
	Yellow and cloudy = not great; rehydration necessary
	Dark yellow/amber = slightly dehydrated
	Dark or orange tint = severely dehydrated

If an athlete does not replace the fluids and electrolytes lost in sweat, a cascade of negative events occurs: a rise in osmolality and a drop in blood pressure, followed by an increase in heart rate. In contrast, if an athlete drinks too much water too quickly, sodium levels will drop, causing cells to swell.

Some athletes don't drink enough water during exercise; it's an afterthought until their workout is over. Others drink too much because coaches and parents excessively direct them to hydrate. Different sports and athletic situations pose different challenges for optimizing hydration. Knowing your individual sweat rate and fluid needs will minimize excessive fluid loss and prevent you from overdrinking during exercise. Advanced methods, such as sweat testing and pee sticks that measure specific gravity, can help personalize hydration needs. Remember, your body doesn't have a water reservoir to store fluid, so you must keep up with your fluid needs on a daily basis, especially around exercise.

Fluid Loss

The majority of your daily fluid output occurs through urination, up to 1,500 milliliters per day. At rest, your body loses water in several ways:

- 60 percent through urination
- 30 percent through skin and respiration (insensible water loss)
- 5 percent through sweat
- 5 percent through bowel movements

During exercise, water can be lost through sweating and from increased aerobic metabolism. Sweating is your body's way of dispersing heat, but it also causes a loss in fluids and electrolytes. We naturally sweat during exercise but at various degrees and volumes. Some athletes can lose up to 67 ounces, or 2 liters, of water per hour during exercise. Sodium loss in athletes ranges from 200 milligrams to more than 2,000 milligrams per liter of sweat. Genetics appear to contribute most to this variability, which is also affected by type of sport, weather conditions, body size/surface area, intensity and duration of exercise, clothing, hydration status, age, health status, and fitness level. One aspect, however, is universal: All active individuals are at risk of dehydration from fluid loss, and those who are physically active in warm environments often fall way short of fluid intake needs because they significantly underestimate sweat and electrolyte losses. Fine-tuning both your daily fluid intake and your exercise fluid intake is a principal strategy to enhance performance and protect your health.

FLUID BALANCE

Fluid balance describes the equilibrium between the fluid input and output in the body that allows metabolic processes to function properly. To maintain this balance, fluids move in and out of cells through a semipermeable cell membrane to maintain equilibrium on both sides. This is called osmosis.

Osmolality is a measure of the concentration of particles in a solution, such as electrolytes and glucose. When your fluid balance gets out of whack, the body responds in two ways:

1. Dehydration: an increase in plasma osmolality triggers the secretion of antidiuretic hormone (ADH), which causes the kidneys to reabsorb water and concentrate urine to be excreted. Plasma osmolality then decreases.

2. Overhydration: ADH secretion is suppressed with a decrease in plasma osmolality, which reduces the quantity of water reabsorbed by the kidneys. More dilute urine is passed to rid excess water in the body. Plasma osmolality increases.

Fluid Intake

Your body gets water in three ways: from drinking water and other fluids (about 60 percent), from food intake (about 30 percent), and from metabolic water produced by cellular respiration (about 10 percent).

The amount of water you drink is primarily regulated by thirst. When your body experiences a water deficit, it moves the fluid from the intracellular compartment over to the extracellular compartment, causing cells to shrink. The reduced cell size tells the brain to initiate drinking and for the kidneys to reduce urine output. When you feel thirsty, it's your body's way of saying you are dehydrated.

When the body contains an excess of water, more fluid reaches the intracellular compartment. The cells absorb the water, your desire to drink water is inhibited, and your kidneys excrete water through urination. Your physical activity, body size, environmental conditions, metabolic rate, sweat loss, age, and exercise duration and intensity all influence how much water or fluid you need. This is why it is difficult to offer a general fluid-intake recommendation that will work for every athlete.

Since the *Dietary Guidelines for Americans* (2015 to 2020) does not provide specific recommendations for water or fluid intake, I follow the guidelines set by the Institute of Medicine in 2004 that recommend about 2.7 liters, or 91 fluid ounces, of total water a day for women, and about 3.7 liters (125 fluid ounces) daily for men. These guidelines include total fluid intake from food and beverages.

Fluid Absorption

The small intestine absorbs a large amount of water from dietary fluid as well as secretions from the salivary glands, pancreas, liver, and even the small intestine itself. By the time water enters the large intestine, roughly 80 percent of fluid absorption has occurred. In the small intestine, water transport occurs in two ways: passively or facilitated. The rate at which food and fluid move from your stomach to your small intestine, called **gastric emptying**, is dependent on the volume and the formulation of ingested contents.

The greater the liquid concentration, the greater the osmolality or movement. For example, when you drink plain water, there's a drive for the water to dilute the blood. Now add in a little sugar with sodium to your beverage, and you can pull a greater amount of water across the small intestine, optimizing rapid absorption. However, consume a **hypertonic** (concentrated) beverage, such as a high-calorie sports drink or soda, and your body has to move water out of the bloodstream and into the gut in order to dilute the high concentration of solutes. For this reason, fluid absorption is optimized when a sports drink is formulated to a concentration that is similar to or less than human blood. These low-osmolality beverages are also known as isotonic or **hypotonic** beverages. To help take away the confusion of sports drinks, I provide several suggestions in chapter 3. Contrary to popular belief, the temperature of a beverage has little effect on fluid absorption except for initiating the craving for a cold versus a warm beverage.

Fluid-Related Issues

Athletes are susceptible to fluid-related issues for many reasons, including but not limited to:

- Poor understanding of fluid needs
- Mismanaged drinking strategies
- Lack of or limited drink opportunities
- Aversion to sports nutrition beverages
- Inability to match excessive sweat rates with fluid intake

Despite the many methods your body has to protect you from overheating, you're still susceptible to several serious and life-threatening health issues in the heat, even if you are drinking a sports drink.

DEHYDRATION

Dehydration occurs when the loss of body mass related to fluid loss occurs at a rate of 1 percent or more. Immediate symptoms include headache, fatigue, and chills. Dehydration can sometimes lead to **cardiovascular drift**, which is the gradual increase in heart rate, independent of effort—common during prolonged activity, especially in the heat. A drop in blood volume leads to hypotension and, if not corrected, the body's organs will no longer receive adequate blood flow, which can cause a stroke, heart attack, kidney failure, or organ failure. If you are exercising in the heat for an hour or more, choose a hypotonic sports drink over water, and drink it every 10 to 15 minutes.

HEAT CRAMPS

Heat cramps are painful, involuntary muscle spasms that typically occur during heavy training in a hot environment. Often the body isn't properly conditioned or an athlete is wearing several layers of clothes. Excessive electrolyte and fluid loss may promote heat cramps. If you have them, stop immediately and don't try to stretch the affected muscle. Lightly massage the area and rehydrate with a sports drink. Do not resume physical activity until the cramp completely goes away.

HEAT EXHAUSTION

Heat exhaustion is the inability of the body to cool itself down when exposed to high temperatures, and it is often accompanied by dehydration, which stops the heart from providing oxygenated blood to the organs and muscles. Symptoms include fatigue, weakness, chills, headache, heavy sweating, dizziness, fainting, nausea, and decreased blood pressure. To avoid heat exhaustion, reduce your effort and gradually increase intensity and duration over a two-week period until you've safely acclimated to the heat. Be sure to include rest breaks during prolonged activity in the heat.

HEATSTROKE

Heatstroke (or sunstroke) occurs when your core body temperature reaches above 104 degrees. Strenuous exercise in (but not limited to) a hot environment is the culprit. During heatstroke, your central nervous system malfunctions and multiple organs fail. This can be fatal if not immediately treated. Symptoms include hyperventilation, altered mental status, dizziness, confusion, inability to walk, loss of balance, collapse, and seizures, and can result in a coma. If it appears that someone you're exercising with is experiencing heat- or sunstroke, move him or her out of the heat and attempt to lower their body temperature with ice packs until emergency personnel arrive.

Excessive water intake can dilute plasma electrolyte concentrations, resulting in dangerously low sodium levels. **Hyponatremia** occurs when the osmotic balance across the blood-brain barrier is disrupted, causing water to enter the brain. Symptoms include nausea, headaches, mental state changes, muscle weakness, seizures, and coma, and the condition can result in death. Athletes who consume little dietary salt, rapidly overconsume plain water, or sweat profusely with inadequate electrolyte intake are at risk. You should design a fluid-intake regimen that prevents overdrinking but optimizes fluids and electrolytes to replenish what you lose in sweat.

Here are a few tips to prevent a heat-related condition:

- Avoid extreme spikes in exercise intensity/volume when training outside.
- Develop a hydration protocol with a sport dietitian to keep up with sweat loss.
- Never exercise when sick. When you return to 80 percent optimal health, slowly resume exercise with low-intensity activity until you feel 100 percent again. As a general rule, if illness symptoms are below the neck, skip exercise. If above the neck, proceed with caution.
- Dress appropriately (light, moisture-wicking layers with SPF protection) and wear sunscreen when training outside.
- Monitor the warning signs of a heat-related illness.

Energy Nutrients

To meet the metabolic demands of your working muscles, your body requires energy in the form of food. When dietary carbohydrates, fats, and proteins break down, you gain fuel for your body. But unlike a car, which continues to drive fast even when the fuel tank is almost empty, your body slows down as you empty your fuel tank.

Carbohydrates are your body's primary energy source, especially during intense or prolonged activity. The amount of carbohydrates stored in your muscles and liver is limited, so you must be strategic with the amount and time of carbohydrate intake relative to exercise.

Stored fat is also a major energy source. Fat releases energy slowly, which makes it a poor fuel source for anaerobic activity but ideal for long aerobic training sessions. The quantity and type of dietary fat that you consume is a hot topic among athletes these days. I'll touch on this topic later in the book.

Protein is not an ideal energy source, but the **amino acids** that make up this nutrient are your body's building blocks. Protein is great at optimizing muscle-adaptation response; it builds and repairs body tissue, bones, and skin. For every gram of carbohydrates or protein, your body receives four calories' worth of energy, whereas one gram of fat generates nine calories.

What, why, and how you eat depends on a host of factors, including ethical and religious beliefs. Medical necessity, food intolerances or allergies, and body-composition goals also influence your diet. Income and food availability shouldn't be overlooked either.

People who want to lose weight through an exercise regimen often limit caloric intake to about 1,500 calories. Some competitive athletes have energy needs of more than 5,000 calories per day. Understanding your specific dietary needs will be addressed in chapter 2.

Carbohydrates

Over the past several years, there has been a backlash against carbohydrates. Because they have been labeled "unhealthy," many athletes now believe that carbs are fattening— *they think* you can't burn fat if you eat carbs. With so much negative attention placed on this one macronutrient, it's easy to believe that carbs will negatively affect performance and body composition. But don't be misled.

Some of the healthiest and fittest people in the world consume a high-carbohydrate diet, with the majority of calories coming from potatoes, rice, legumes, and vegetables.

Carbohydrates provide the best source of energy, particularly for intermittent sports, endurance activities, and high-intensity exercise. This fuel assists fat metabolism, delays fatigue, and supports the central nervous system. Adequate carbohydrate intake can safeguard your glycogen storage and protein stores and support blood sugar levels during exercise, helping you sustain energy during your hard workouts and protect your immune system.

The research on carbohydrates may look conflicting, but if you prioritize real, wholesome, nutrient-dense sources of food instead of processed, refined, nutrient-poor sources, you, too, can experience great performance without sabotaging your health or body composition goals.

Carb intake should be strategically adjusted around exercise sessions, competitions, and off-season training. However, athletes and fitness enthusiasts should maintain a healthy relationship with carbs all year long.

SIMPLE CARBOHYDRATES

There are two types of simple sugars: **monosaccharides** and **disaccharides**. Within each classification are the various sugars found in plant and animal foods.

Monosaccharides include:

Glucose, also known as dextrose, is a sugar that occurs naturally in food and also lives in our blood. Insulin is required for it to be metabolized in the body. Glucose can also be produced through non-carbohydrate substrates such as lactate, amino acids and fatty acids to help maintain blood glucose levels. This is also known as **gluconeogenesis**.

Fructose is found in fruit and honey, and doesn't require insulin for metabolization. It's absorbed from the small intestine and transported to the liver, where roughly 50 percent of it is converted to glucose.

Galactose is mostly found in dairy products. When combined with glucose, it forms the milk sugar lactose. Galactose converts into glucose for energy metabolism.

Combining two monosaccharide molecules forms a disaccharide, or double sugar. Disaccharides always contain glucose:

Sucrose (glucose and fructose) is commonly found in white sugar, cane sugar, brown sugar, sorghum, maple syrup, honey, corn syrup, and high-fructose corn syrup (HFCS). Honey is sweeter than table sugar because of its high fructose content, about 40 percent. HFCS contains about 42 percent fructose. Agave nectar contains anywhere from 56 percent to 90 percent fructose.

Lactose (glucose and galactose) is the natural sugar found in milk. People who have lactose intolerance have trouble digesting this sugar because they don't have adequate amounts of the enzyme lactase, which is needed for that process. Lactose-free beverages include soy, almond, coconut, and rice milks. Buyer beware, though: Many milk alternatives contain added sugar.

Maltose (glucose and glucose) is also known as malt sugar, and is produced in the breakdown of starch. It can be found in beer, cereals, bread, and, of course, in malted milkshakes.

Sugary foods are pleasurable and convenient, but they're also addictive and easy to consume in excess. Table sugar has 16 calories per teaspoon. Once your body absorbs sugar, it can't distinguish the original sugar source. But your body does digest sugar types in different ways. The small intestine produces enzymes to break down disaccharides into monosaccharides, which can then be absorbed by the body without further breakdown. This is why sports drinks with glucose and fructose are ideal: The sugars are absorbed relatively easily. When reviewing food labels, pay attention to the amount of added sugar. Women should limit added sugar to 6 teaspoons a day, and men should limit it to 9 teaspoons. This doesn't include the nutrition consumed during workouts or natural sugars found in foods like raisins, carrots, and bananas. Consuming naturally sweet foods like fruit or plain yogurt when you crave a treat can help lower your added-sugar consumption.

COMPLEX CARBOHYDRATES

Complex carbs are also known as **polysaccharides**. Three main types exist:

1. **Starch** is the storage form of carbohydrates in plants. It is found abundantly in seeds, corn, and grains, as well as in peas, beans, potatoes, and root vegetables. The starch in these plant sources can be broken down into two forms:

    Amylose: Found in basmati rice, long-grain rice, barley, corn, oats, potatoes, and bananas. These foods break down and digest slowly.

    Amylopectin: Found in jasmine rice, sushi (or glutinous) rice, and Russet Burbank potatoes. These foods digest and absorb rapidly.

2. **Glycogen** is the storage polysaccharide found in mammalian muscle and the liver. Approximately 65 percent of glycogen is water. Muscle glycogen acts as a major energy source for active muscles.

3. **Fiber** is classified as a nonstarch polysaccharide and exists exclusively in plants. It makes up the structure of fruit leaves, stems, roots, seeds, and skins. Fiber can be divided into two categories:

    Water-soluble fibers: Pectin (fruit, vegetables, legumes, potatoes), and guar gum (oats, legumes, barley, brown rice, peas, carrots, fruit)

    Water-insoluble fibers: Hemicellulose (cereal grains), cellulose (vegetables), lignins (woody plants), mucilage (plant extracts), and gums (leguminous seed plants, seaweed extracts, microbial gums)

    Fiber slows digestion, promotes satiety, and provides "bulk" to food residue in the intestines. The recommended daily amount of fiber is 20 to 35 grams. Following this dietary guideline can help reduce your risk of obesity, diabetes, hypertension, and heart disease. Fiber may also improve mental clarity. Increased water-soluble fiber is known to reduce serum cholesterol to improve heart health. Unfortunately, the Western diet is very low in natural plant fiber, and this could be contributing to the rise of gut- and immune system–related issues. Although fiber is important in the athlete's diet, consuming too much fiber too close to exercise time can irritate the gut, increasing the risk of gastro-intestinal (GI) problems such as nausea and diarrhea. I will discuss nutrient timing more in part 2.

SLOW AND FAST CARBOHYDRATES

The body doesn't digest and absorb carbohydrates at the same rate. The **glycemic index (GI)** is a value given to foods based on the rate at which they cause an increase in blood glucose levels. Foods can be ranked as low-, medium-, or high-glycemic. Foods ranked low on the scale release glucose slowly and steadily into the bloodstream. Foods ranked high on the scale release glucose rapidly into the bloodstream. When a carbohydrate is combined with fat or fiber, digestion is slowed along with the glucose response.

The GI value only represents the type of carbohydrate. The **glycemic load (GL)** combines both the quantity and quality of carbohydrates. The GI doesn't take into account the amount of carbohydrates in a given food, so the GL is a good indicator of how a carbohydrate will affect blood sugar levels. Interestingly, the GI doesn't consider carbohydrate classification, such as "simple" (mono- and disaccharides) or "complex" (starch and fiber). As an example, a potato (plant starch) has a higher GI than an apple (fructose).

Glycemic index of food (glucose = 100)

LOW (55 or LESS)	MEDIUM (55-69)	HIGH (70+)
100% whole wheat	Rye bread, pita bread	White bread, bagel
Steel-cut oats, oat bran	Quick oats	Cornflakes
Barley, bulgur	Brown, wild, and basmati rice	Instant oats
Sweet potatoes	Couscous	Russet potatoes
Legumes	Orange juice	Pretzels
Nonstarchy veggies	Jam	Rice cakes
Carrots	Honey	Saltine crackers
Apples	Pineapple	Watermelon
Milk	Muesli	White rice
Fructose	Corn	Rice milk

Understanding the GI can help you fine-tune your intake of dietary carbohydrates. For example, a carbohydrate with a high glycemic index, such as saltine crackers, may sit better in the gut before an intense workout than a low glycemic food, such as steel-cut oats, would. Interestingly, the effects of consuming low-, medium-, or high-glycemic foods around workouts are inconsistent related to performance. Athletes are encouraged to prioritize high-fiber, slow-digesting carbohydrates as part of a healthy diet. It's also good practice, however, to let your experiences and preferences, as well as food availability, dictate the type of carbohydrates to consume before, during, and after exercise and competitions.

CARBOHYDRATE REQUIREMENTS

To optimize performance during prolonged or high-intensity activity, you must have adequate glycogen stored in your muscles and liver, and glucose in your blood. All are critical to maintaining energy when you exercise. Carbohydrate recommendations vary based on body weight and training load, and carbs should be consumed throughout the day to promote consistent fuel availability.

Carbohydrate recommendations based on workout volume/intensity

TYPE OF ACTIVITY	RECOMMENDED CARB INTAKE
Low intensity/very light activity	3-5 grams/kilograms/day
Moderate intensity, 1 hour per day	5-7g/kg/d
Moderate to high intensity/duration, about 1-3 hours per day	6-10g/kg/d
High intensity/duration, 4-5 hours per day	8-12g/kg/d

1 lb = 2.2kg

For an athlete to meet specific carbohydrate recommendations, energy intake must balance energy expenditure. For example, take a 140-pound athlete who trains for two hours a day and intentionally restricts calories to only 1,500 a day. Even if 50 percent of those calories come from carbohydrates, the athlete will fall short of their minimum carbohydrate needs because of the low-calorie diet. A well-planned, energy-sufficient diet is crucial for maintaining adequate energy storage for training.

Here are some common foods that have 25 grams of carbohydrates:

- 2 fig cookies
- 2-ounce English muffin
- 2 slices bread
- ½ cup rice
- ½ cup cooked pasta
- 2 cups milk
- 6 ounces plain yogurt
- ½ cup black beans
- 17 mini pretzels
- ½ medium potato with skin
- 2 cups fresh strawberries
- 1 large orange
- 1 medium banana

AMINO ACIDS

A protein molecule is a nitrogenous organic compound consisting of long chains of linked building blocks called amino acids. Peptide bonds link the amino acids to create chains of many different forms and combinations. The body requires 20 different amino acids. Nine of them can't be synthesized in the body, so we must obtain them from our diet. These are called essential amino acids. Eleven are nonessential, meaning they're synthesized from other compounds already inside the body. As an athlete, you may have heard of **branch chain amino acids (BCAAs)**. These three essential amino acids play many roles during exercise performance (see chapter 6). Proteins can be further classified as complete or incomplete, depending on the quality. Complete proteins, typically found in animal sources, contain all the essential amino acids in the quantity necessary to fulfill daily bodily functions. Incomplete proteins, found in plants, lack one or more essential amino acids. Eating a variety of proteins will ensure that you're meeting all of your amino acid needs.

Protein

Our society is currently obsessed with protein. Without a doubt, protein is a powerful macronutrient. It's a component in every cell in the body. You can find protein in your hair, skin, and nails. It's used to construct and repair tissue, build strong bones and muscles, and make enzymes, hormones, and other chemicals. However, there's a tendency for athletes and fitness enthusiasts to rely heavily on supplemental forms of protein, such as powder mixes or bars, instead of real food.

There are several factors that can affect individual protein needs. For example, a woman who attends a weekly yoga class will have a different protein requirement than a woman training for a power-lifting competition. And people who are hospitalized may need to consume a specific amount of protein for optimal healing. Here are a few other examples of factors that can influence protein needs:

- High levels of physical activity
- Endurance- and strength-focused physical activity
- Age-related health conditions (i.e., **osteoporosis**)
- Burn-related health conditions
- Restricting calories to foster weight loss
- Health conditions such as cancer and kidney disease

There's a good chance that you're already sufficiently meeting your unique protein needs, but you could be far off. Much of this depends on your physical activity routine and dietary choices, so it's important to reassess your dietary protein intake every week to see if you need to add more to your diet.

PROTEIN SOURCES

There are many different protein options available. Depending on where you live, some are more readily available and consumed than others. Protein sources include animals, plants, and engineered foods. Common animal sources include meat, poultry, seafood, eggs, and dairy. Plant sources of protein can be found in legumes such as beans, lentils and peas, and soy products such as tempeh and tofu. Nuts, edamame, seeds, and grains contain protein as well. Engineered sources include powders, bars, and factory-made "high-protein" foods such as cereals and breads.

Animal protein sources make up roughly two-thirds of the dietary protein intake in a standard diet, but whole grains, soy, and legumes are also excellent sources of protein. You don't have to be a vegan to consume plant-based proteins. The nutrients commonly found in animal protein include:

- Vitamin B12
- Omega-3 fatty acids
- Zinc
- Iron

Heme iron is found only in meat, poultry, shellfish, and fish. Non-heme iron is found in plant and animal foods. Heme iron is more easily absorbed than non-heme iron. For example, about 20 to 30 percent of the iron found in beef is absorbed into the bloodstream, while just 5 to 12 percent of the iron found in spinach is absorbed. This can cause some athletes to be at risk of iron-deficiency issues depending on protein quality and consumption.

Nutrients commonly found in plant proteins include:

- Magnesium
- Phytonutrients
- Folate
- Calcium

Protein supplements have a long history in sports. Athletes commonly reach for them as meal substitutes, to increase energy, promote weight gain or loss, repair muscle, and boost performance and recovery.

With an array of available protein powders and bars, the primary protein ingredient will likely be whey, casein, soy, or vegan-based (as in brown rice or pea). All proteins contain amino acids but not all proteins are considered equal. Both whey and casein are derived from milk. They're essentially the by-products of making cheese. Whey is a complete protein and comes in two forms: concentrate or isolate. Whey concentrate contains 70 to 80 percent protein, with low amounts of lactose and fat, while whey isolate contains 90 to 95 percent protein and almost no fat and lactose. Although isolate contains more protein, concentrate is no less superior if it fits your budget and you like the taste.

Whey empties from the stomach rather quickly, whereas casein provides a slower release of amino acids. Soy contains a low amount of the **anabolic** trigger **leucine**, which makes it inferior to whey but a suitable option for plant-based athletes. Vegan powders lack all essential amino acids; however, quinoa would make an excellent protein powder because it contains leucine, lysine, and methionine—similar to milk. It's true that protein supplements are convenient for increasing or quickly consuming protein, but they should not be viewed as a replacement for real food.

PROTEIN REQUIREMENTS

Your body doesn't store protein like it does carbohydrates and fats, so be sure to distribute your protein intake throughout the day. A total of 25 to 30 grams of protein per meal is a good range. The **daily reference intake (DRI)** is set at 0.8 grams of protein per each kilogram of body weight. This amounts to about 54 grams protein for a 150-pound individual, equivalent to four sausage links, one Greek yogurt, and two eggs. I feel this is too low for athletes. Instead, I agree with the Academy of Nutrition and Dietetics, which recommends that athletes aim for 1.2 to 2 grams of protein per each kilogram of body weight. Only 5 to 15 percent of total energy expenditure during exercise comes from protein, so if your body is using protein as a direct fuel source, you'll lose muscle instead of gaining it.

As an easy reference, there are about 7 grams of protein in 1 ounce of cooked meat. Here are some excellent go-to protein foods:

- 3.5 ounces chicken breast – 30 grams
- 3 ounces canned tuna – 25 grams
- ½ cup tofu – 20 grams
- ½ cup cottage cheese – 15 grams
- 1 ounce cheese – 8 grams
- 1 cup milk – 8 grams
- 1 cup yogurt – 8 to 17 grams
- 2 tablespoons peanut butter – 8 grams
- ¼ cup almonds – 8 grams
- ¼ cup flaxseeds – 8 grams
- 1 large egg – 6 grams

Fat

There is a lot of confusion about dietary fat in our body-image–obsessed society. The notion that "fat makes you fat" has controlled the popular mindset for decades. Thankfully, nutrition research has evolved to prove that dietary fat, in the right amounts and types, is important for a healthy, functioning body.

Because of its slow digestion time, fat promotes satiety, delays the onset of hunger pangs, and can reduce cravings and overeating. Fat also acts as an energy reserve,

PROTEIN QUALITY

Protein quality describes the rate at which protein is absorbed into the body and the quantity of essential amino acids. There are two notable methods for determining the quality of protein food sources.

1. **Biological value (BV):** This analyzes the body's ability to digest, absorb, and excrete proteins. Urine and feces are tested for nitrogen levels and are compared with whole food. The drawback is that nitrogen retention during exercise or fasting can compromise results.

2. **Protein digestibility–corrected (per National Library of Medicine) amino acid score (PDCAAS):** This is a method of determining protein quality by comparing the amino acid profile of a specific protein against a standard amino acid profile, with the highest score being 1.0. This means that after protein digestion, the food provides 100% or more of the essential amino acids required per unit of protein. Here are the protein digestibility percentages of some common types of food:

   - Eggs – 100%
   - Milk –100%
   - Ground beef – 92%
   - Soy – 91% (limiting AA methionine, cysteine)
   - Corn – 52% (limiting AA lysine)
   - Wheat – 42% (limiting AA lysine)

provides fat-soluble vitamins, supplies essential fatty acids, offers thermal insulation, and protects vital organs.

We all love ice cream, potato chips, and cheese, but when consumed in excess, these high-fat foods may increase the risk of weight gain metabolic disease. One way to keep from overconsuming them is to prioritize fat from natural sources, primarily plants. But I'm here to say that there's no need to fear fat in your diet.

SATURATED FATS

Saturated fats occur primarily in animal products, such as beef, bacon, egg yolks, cheese, full-fat dairy, and butter. They remain solid at room temperature. In the plant kingdom, coconut oil, palm kernel oil, and vegetable shortening contain saturated fats. Often called the "bad" fats, they're linked to increased **cholesterol** levels and

KETOGENIC DIET

The ketogenic diet was originally developed in the 1920s as a drug-free way to treat epilepsy in children. The chemicals produced as a result of the diet, ketones and decanoic acid, were found to help control seizures in some people with epilepsy.

The diet—low-carb, high-fat—sounds attractive. After all, people who adopt this diet are advised to eat cream, butter, oil, and naturally fatty foods. In a ketogenic diet, roughly 75 percent of calories come from fats, 20 percent from protein, and 5 percent from carbohydrates. Carbohydrates are restricted to fewer than 50 grams per day. This is equal to 1 cup milk and 1½ cups cereal.

Under normal physiological conditions, glucose is the brain's major energy source. Under ketosis, the body must find an alternative energy source for the brain. That's when the liver kicks in and forms ketone bodies.

Complications from a ketogenic diet can include impaired metabolism, hypoglycemia, increased sickness/injury, hormonal disturbance, dehydration, nutrient deficiencies, reduced capacity to utilize carbs, and central nervous system fatigue. Although current literature has shown metabolic adaptions among endurance athletes on high-fat, carbohydrate-restricted diets, the performance and health benefits aren't consistent enough for me to endorse this diet for athletes.

heart disease. With much conflicting information on saturated fats, it's recommended to eat them in moderation, as part of a well-planned, whole-foods diet. Remember, your diet consists of many puzzle pieces, so combining a hardboiled egg or a cup of full-fat yogurt with a bowl of oatmeal can make for a healthy, satisfying, and performance-boosting meal.

UNSATURATED FATS

Unsaturated fats are typically plant-based and tend to liquefy at room temperature. The two main types are:

Monounsaturated fats (omega-9s). A diet rich in monounsaturated fats can help keep blood cholesterol levels down. They're considered essential. Avocado, almond, pecan, cashew, and olive oils are excellent sources.

Polyunsaturated fats (omega-3s and omega-6s). Your body can't make polyunsaturated fats, which makes them essential. Benefits include building cell membranes, assisting in blood clotting and muscle movement, and reducing inflammation.

Flaxseed, anchovies, catfish, mackerel, salmon, tuna, and shrimp are good sources of omega-3s, while pumpkin seeds and soybean, safflower, and corn oils are full of omega-6s.

Trans fats in food are also known as *partially hydrogenated* oils. They are manufactured and don't occur in nature. The chemical process converts an unsaturated oil into a saturated fat, which can remain solid at room temperature. Artificial trans fats are easy to use and inexpensive, and they preserve the shelf life of many foods. Margarine is made of trans fats.

Studies have shown that this type of fat raises bad cholesterol and increases the risk of heart disease and stroke. As of June 2018, the **Food and Drug Administration (FDA)** has banned the addition of partially hydrogenated fats to processed foods.

FAT REQUIREMENTS

Recommended daily intake of fat is set to at least 1 g/kg/d. Too much or too little fat can be harmful to health and performance. Although no particular fat should be deemed "bad," certain fats should be consumed more regularly than others. Give priority to unsaturated fatty acids for ongoing support of heart benefits. Be sure to keep your kitchen stocked with these go-to unsaturated fats as part of a heart-healthy athletic diet:

- Olive oil
- Canola oil
- Almonds
- Avocado
- Peanut butter
- Cashews
- Walnuts
- Sunflower seeds
- Pumpkin seeds
- Low-fat dairy
- Fatty fish
- Flaxseeds
- Chia seeds

The following foods contain high amounts of saturated fats, so make sure to consume them in moderation:

- Coconut oil
- Butter
- Whole eggs
- Cream cheese
- Cheese
- Beef

Vitamins and Minerals

Unlike **macronutrients** (carbohydrates, protein, and fat), **micronutrients** are needed in much smaller quantities. But don't underestimate these powerful nutrients—macronutrient metabolism requires micronutrients to be present.

OMEGA-3S AND OMEGA-6S

Omega-3 and **omega-6 fatty acids** are polyunsaturated fatty acids. There's strong evidence that omega-3 fatty acids may improve heart health, lower **triglycerides,** improve endothelial function, and reduce inflammation.

- **Omega-3s** include **alpha-linolenic acid (ALA), eicosapentaenoic acid (EPA),** and **docosahexaenoic acid (DHA).**

- **Omega-6s** include **linoleic acid** and **arachidonic acid**.

Common food sources for these polyunsaturated fats include:

- **ALA:** canola oil, flaxseeds, chia seeds, English walnuts, soybeans

- **DHA/EPA:** Atlantic salmon, Atlantic herring, canned sardines, trout, oysters, fish oil, krill oil (synthesized by microalgae, not by the fish)

- **Linoleic acid:** flaxseeds, hemp seeds, grapeseed oil, pistachios, acai

- **Arachidonic acid:** poultry, eggs, beef, fish

ALA and linoleic acid must be obtained from the diet since they are essential fatty acids. ALA can be converted into EPA and DHA, but the conversion in the liver is limited.

For athletes, omega-3s may improve blood vessel function, reduce inflammation, and improve decision-making and mood. It's inconclusive whether fish oil supplements can improve athletic performance. Some research suggests that high doses of omega-3 supplements may increase oxidative stress and place athletes at risk for a suppressed immune system.

If dietary micronutrients are inadequate, your body can't function. **Vitamins** and **minerals** have many important functions. They provide energy metabolism, protect against oxidative damage, and support your immune system. Exercise places extreme stress on metabolic pathways. Athletes with insufficient energy intake or impaired absorption are at risk of a micronutrient deficiency. No single food can supply all of the nutrients you need in appropriate amounts, so be sure to eat a variety of foods to boost your health and performance.

Vitamins

Vitamins are organic compounds classified by their solubility: fat-soluble and water-soluble. Fat-soluble vitamins require fat for absorption and are stored in the liver and fatty tissue. They eliminate slowly from the body and can cause toxicity if consumed in excess. In contrast, water-soluble vitamins dissolve effortlessly in water and aren't stored in the body. These vitamins are easily broken down and excreted in urine, so constant replenishment is needed. Vitamins don't contain calories; they can't boost energy. But they do work with your diet to turn food into energy.

Vitamin Type	Food Sources	Function
Water-Soluble Vitamins		
Thiamin (B1)	Wheat germ, brewer's yeast, oysters, peanuts, green peas, raisins, enriched grains	Carbohydrate metabolism
Riboflavin (B2)	Organ meats, milk, cheese, oily fish, eggs, dark leafy greens	Contributes to energy metabolism
Niacin (B3)	Beef, pork, chicken, wheat flour, eggs, milk	Assists in nervous system functioning and food metabolism
Pantothenic acid (B5)	Eggs, whole grains, fortified cereals, meat	Plays an essential role in cellular metabolism and energy production
Pyridoxin (B6)	Liver, chicken, bananas, potatoes, spinach	Helps metabolize amino acids; releases energy from food
Biotin (B7)	Kidney, liver, eggs, dried fruit	Coenzyme in the synthesis of fat, B vitamins, and amino aids
Folic acid (B9)	Dark leafy greens, dry beans, peas, grains	Helps with cell growth; forms red and white blood cells
Cobalamin (B12)	Eggs, milk, meat, fortified cereals, nutritional yeast	Assists in the function of the brain and nervous system
Vitamin C	Brussels sprouts, broccoli, bell peppers, kiwis, oranges, papayas, guavas	Helps with growth and repair of tissue

Vitamin Type	Food Sources	Function
Fat-Soluble Vitamins		
Vitamin A	Carrots, broccoli, tomatoes, liver, milk	Boosts vision, skin, and the immune system
Vitamin D	Oily fish, liver, eggs, fortified foods, bread, milk	Provides strength to bones and teeth
Vitamin E	Plant oils, nuts, seeds, wheat germ	Works as an antioxidant; supports the immune system
Vitamin K	Dark leafy greens, cabbage, green tea, alfalfa, oats, cauliflower	Crucial to fetus growth and blood clotting

Minerals

Minerals are inorganic elements that exist as solids. They're classified as trace or major. Trace minerals are needed in small amounts, less than 20 milligrams per day. Major minerals are needed in large amounts, more than 100 milligrams per day. Similar to vitamins, low mineral intakes may result in a deficiency. Athletes who eliminate one or more food groups from their diet, eat poorly, or partake in extreme weight-loss practices are at the greatest risk of poor micronutrient intakes.

Mineral Type	Food Sources	Function
Major		
Calcium	Milk, cheese, dark leafy greens, legumes, fortified cereals	Stimulates muscle and nerve function; crucial for bone-building
Phosphorus	Milk, cheese, yogurt, meat, poultry, grains, fish	Promotes DNA synthesis, acid-base balance, and energy transfer
Potassium	Dark leafy greens, cantaloupes, lima beans, potatoes, bananas, milk	Facilitates fluid volume; helps lower blood pressure; conducts nerve impulses and muscle contractions; plays critical role in cardiac functioning
Sodium	Table salt (sodium chloride), cured meats, processed cheese, packaged foods	Maintains fluid volume outside of cells; plays a key role in normal nerve and muscle functions

Mineral Type	Food Sources	Function
Magnesium	Whole grains, dark leafy greens, nuts, seeds, legumes	Regulates blood glucose levels; helps maintain muscle function
Trace		
Iron	Eggs, lean meats, legumes, whole grains, dark leafy greens, black-strap molasses, tofu	Transports and stores oxygen; involved in ATP synthesis and red blood cell formation
Zinc	Oysters, red meat, poultry, beans, nuts, seafood, whole grains, forti-fied cereals, dairy	Energy metabolism
Copper	Beef liver, sunflower seeds, lentils, dried apricots, dark chocolate, sweet potatoes	Helps produce enzymes; plays a role in iron metabolism
Selenium	Seafood, meats, grains, mush-rooms, asparagus	Antioxidant agent; regulates thyroid hormones
Iodine	Iodized salt, marine fish and shellfish, dairy, strawberries, cantaloupes	Component of thyroid hormones
Chromium	Legumes, cereals, organ meats, fats, vegetable oils, beans, black tea	Promotes glucose uptake; main-tains glucose levels

Vitamin and Mineral Supplements

Many athletes rely on multivitamins to make up for unhealthy eating habits, boost performance, and reduce the risk of injury or sickness. Individual vitamin and mineral supplements may be useful, especially if you've identified a nutrient hole in your diet and real food won't fill the gap. However, remember that multivitamins contain varying amounts of nutrients and aren't well-regulated. That's why food is best to help you meet your nutritional needs. Nutrient deficiencies often occur when energy intake is insufficient relative to energy expenditure, so athletes need to be mindful of how their daily diet influences the amount of vitamins and minerals they consume. A "plate not pill" approach saves money and remains the most practical way to optimize health and performance.

Supplements come in a variety of forms: tablets, liquids, powders, bars, and capsules. Some of the most sought-after vitamin and mineral supplements include iron, B12, vitamin D, calcium, multivitamins, and **antioxidants** like vitamins C, E, and Q10. Some supplements are problematic to health and performance. A review in the *Journal of Physiology* showed no strong evidence that antioxidant supplements, such as vitamins C and E, improve performance or health. Furthermore, high-dose antioxidants may prevent important training adaptations, such as creating new muscle mitochondria, muscle growth, and improving insulin sensitivity. In addition, supplements contain multiple ingredients, making it difficult to know or predict the efficacy and safety of your desired product. With so much concern over supplements containing banned substances (which will cause an athlete to fail a drug test), it's best to obtain your vitamins and minerals from food—just like nature intended. If you're considering a supplement, first consult with a board-certified sports dietitian.

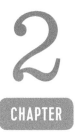

CHAPTER

Components of an Optimal Diet

When it comes to sports success, diet is a big piece of the puzzle that many athletes struggle to appreciate and master. A healthy diet designed to optimize performance doesn't have to be confusing. Despite the strong relationship between good nutrition habits and athletic success, many athletes disregard their diet in favor of training harder or longer. In reality, it is only when you supply your body with optimal nutrition that you can perform at optimal levels.

People have strong opinions about nutrition, and it can be easy to fall victim to extreme dogmatic mantras. But the truth is that every human being responds differently to different foods. It's impossible to prescribe a one-size-fits-all diet plan. Having said that, the essential component of a healthy diet is very simple: Prioritize whole foods while minimizing processed foods.

In this chapter, you'll begin to personalize your diet so it works for your health and fitness goals. Say goodbye to food rules and dieting as you learn realistic, healthy, and sustainable eating practices, tailored to your physical, psychological, cultural, financial, and social needs.

Hydration

As discussed in chapter 1, the first step to optimizing performance is mastering your daily hydration needs to maintain proper body functions. Fluids are critical to optimal health. They replenish what has been lost through normal physiological processes, such as respiration, sweating, and urination. Ironically, in many athletic settings, water is consistently underconsumed even though the need for it is often overstressed.

The benefits of good hydration practices during exercise include:

- Lower heart rate
- Higher skin blood flow
- Lower core body temperature
- Lower perceived exertion
- Improved skills and concentration
- Reduced incidence of gastrointestinal issues
- Higher **cardiac output** (amount of blood pumped by the heart each minute)
- Higher **stroke volume** (volume of blood pumped from the left ventricle of the heart in one contraction)
- Improved muscle and joint functioning
- Improved digestion and gastric emptying
- Improved performance

The golden rule is no longer that you should drink eight 8-ounce glasses of water a day. Fluid needs vary based on physical activity, environment, age, body size, body composition, and gender. For example, an active teenager may need to consume 64 ounces of fluid just to support a single training session. Based on current literature, the appropriate daily fluid intake goal is 91 ounces for women and 125 ounces for men. Because beverages supply more than 20 percent of the calories in the typical American diet, choose water instead of sugar-sweetened drinks such as fruit juices, sports drinks, sodas, and alcohol. Diarrhea, vomiting, extreme sweat rates, the use of laxatives and diuretics, dieting, and illness also contribute to excessive water loss from the body, and this can compromise health and performance.

Dehydration and Performance

As you learned in chapter 1, every cell, tissue, and organ in your body consists of water and needs water to function. Fifty to 65 percent of your body weight is water. To understand how crucial water is to your body's function, let's take a look at what happens when dehydration occurs.

More than half of your blood volume consists of blood plasma, with water making up about 92 percent of plasma. As the amount of circulating blood—also known as **blood volume**—decreases, your body compensates by retaining more sodium in the blood. As your blood becomes more concentrated and thicker, your blood pressure increases. In turn, your heart works harder because the amount of blood it can pump per beat is reduced. The cardiac output is altered, causing a rise in heart rate and making blood more difficult to circulate. Consequently, blood flow to the working muscles is reduced and performance becomes compromised.

A notable sign of dehydration is when a once-sustainable effort becomes incredibly difficult to maintain. Because of the tremendous stress athletes place on their cardio system, they may also complain of postural hypotension symptoms, such as feeling dizzy, lightheaded, or nauseated. They could also struggle with focus, motivation, and skills.

Dehydration can also bring on the chills. This may sound counterintuitive, but it's because less blood is reaching your skin. As your body retains more heat, this can lead to overheating and slower emptying of nutrients from the gut. All of this may occur with only a 2 percent loss of body weight during exercise. As fluid loss increases, the effects on performance and health become even more damaging. Athletes who participate in endurance, high-intensity, intermittent, and stop-and-go sports are likely to struggle with meeting hydration needs during activity. Wearing heavy clothing and using heavy equipment only exacerbates the issue.

You may not feel thirsty during a workout, but it's absolutely necessary to hydrate while you exercise. You can easily lose more than 1.5 liters of body water before you feel thirsty, which demonstrates that your thirst mechanism is not a reliable indicator of how much water you really need. Moreover, athletes who wait too long to drink have a habit of overdrinking plain water, which can dilute the sodium content of the blood and lead to a sloshy stomach.

To optimize cardiovascular and thermoregulatory functions, subscribe to a comprehensive fluid-replacement program. Identify the best beverages to consume and plan your fluid intake—frequency and volume—around and during exercise.

Thinking About What You Drink

The human body relies on safe water as an essential component of healthy living. With so many popular beverage options available, plain water is still the ideal fluid to consume daily. Water is free of sugar. It doesn't contain caffeine, calories, food dyes, or artificial ingredients, and it's refreshingly good for you. With a growing number of bottled drinks on the market, the type of drink you choose can influence your health and performance more than you think. There is a time and place for sports drinks, and even the occasional soda or glass of wine, but water will always reign when it comes to the health and wellness of your body.

Cities invest millions of dollars to provide the public with pure and safe drinking water. Although tap water often gets a bad rap—the residents of Flint, Michigan, have a lot to say on this subject—it's often just as good as what you find in a bottle, and without the plastic. To find out if your tap water is safe, go to the Environmental Protection Agency's website (EPA.gov) and check out the local drinking water information page.

Below is a quick summary of the kinds of water available:

- **Purified water** is produced by distillation, deionization, reverse **osmosis**, and carbon filtration. Overall impurity levels can't exceed 10 parts per million, and the water is free of contaminants or chemicals.
- **Spring water** is water that flows to the surface of the earth and is collected only at the spring.
- **Alkaline water** is less acidic than tap water and contains compounds that are believed to neutralize acids in your bloodstream. Because the body already tightly regulates pH levels, there's little evidence that water with a high pH is healthier than tap water.

CARBONATED WATER

If you crave a refreshing drink, carbonated water is a great alternative to soda. It lacks the calories and added sugar of soda but still provides a naturally sweet and revitalizing taste. There is some misconception that carbonated drinks can weaken bones and cause tooth decay. As long as your bubbly beverage is free of citric acid, sugar, and phosphorus, there's little risk to your health. Carbonation occurs when water is infused with carbon dioxide, giving it a slightly acidic pH. The trendy SodaStream kit is an example of an at-home seltzer water carbonation system that comes with a reusable BPA-free bottle.

In Europe, seltzer, sparkling, and mineral waters are extremely popular. The primary drawbacks of carbonated water are bloating and gas. Drink any type of carbonated beverage too quickly, and you may experience discomfort in your gut.

TEA

If you're a tea drinker in a coffee-obsessed world, you'll be delighted to hear that there are minimal downsides to drinking tea. With far less caffeine than coffee, and rich in flavonoids and antioxidants, tea is highly praised for its many health benefits. Research from the journal *Current Medicinal Chemistry* shows that green, black, and white teas contain properties that can help fight free radicals and reduce the risk of heart disease and cancer. Popular herbal teas include ginkgo biloba, ginseng, rosehip, chamomile,

WATER BOTTLES

Nearly one billion people in the developing world lack access to safe drinking water. For those who live without clean water sources, the multibillion-dollar water industry makes it easy to take accessible, clean water for granted. Although water in a bottle can be a healthier choice, there's growing concern about the environmental footprint of bottled water. According to *National Geographic*, nearly 91 percent of all plastic bottles don't get recycled. Instead, they accumulate in a plastic-filled landfill or in the ocean. When plastic bottles end up in the sea, animals, the environment, and the land are negatively affected. What's more, plastic bottles contain bisphenol A (BPA) and phthalates to make the container clear, hard, and flexible. But both components have shown to be endocrine disruptors and are linked to a host of damaging health issues.

Make a positive environmental impact: Buy a BPA-free reusable plastic bottle. Even better, choose a reusable bottle made of glass or stainless steel. (Note: If you are allergic to nickel, avoid stainless steel.) Then you can stay hydrated from the tap or a water fountain. If you're concerned about your tap water, get a water-quality report or invest in a water filter. And of course, recycle whenever possible.

echinacea, and hibiscus, and they may boost immunity, assist in weight loss, control appetite, promote restful sleep, and reduce stress.

While herbal tea enthusiasts claim benefits, tea is not a magic bullet. It should be incorporated into an overall healthy diet. Instant teas lack nutrients, contain very little tea, and have high amounts of sugar or artificial sweeteners. Some alternative medicine professionals believe tea holds properties that can fight or prevent cancer, but research has yet to prove this. In some cases, consuming tea is discouraged. Green tea should be avoided if you take blood-thinning medications such as aspirin, ibuprofen, naproxen, and warfarin because of negative interactions with these medications.

COFFEE

Coffee is a global addiction, a staple morning beverage. Coffee connoisseurs will agree that it's the best, and only, way to start the day. Whether you like it, love it, need it, or can't handle it, coffee is one of the most commonly consumed beverages in the world, second only to water. In 2016, the World Health Organization removed coffee from the list of potentially carcinogenic foods, and it is now considered "probably harmless and possibly healthy." If you don't like coffee, there's no need to start drinking it, and if you drink it, there's no need to give it up. Coffee is a central nervous stimulant, though, so drink it in

CAFFEINE

Caffeine naturally occurs in coffee beans and other botanical sources such as chai, oolong, black, and green teas. The caffeine content varies, from 80 to 150 milligrams in an eight-ounce coffee to 30 to 80 milligrams in a serving of black or green tea (three-minute brew time).

Caffeine can also be made in laboratories and added to energy drinks, sports nutrition products, and dietary supplements. Synthetic caffeine will absorb through the digestive tract much faster than naturally occurring caffeine. Check ingredient labels for these commonly consumed stimulant drugs: bitter orange (*citrus aurantium*), green tea extract, caffeine anhydrous, kola nut, cola, coffee extract, yerba mate, and guarana.

Caffeine is a drug. Its side effects include insomnia, restlessness, stomach upset, nausea, increased heart and breathing rates, and anxiety. Its impact on the cardiovascular system can't be overstated; there's always a risk of death when caffeine is improperly used or overconsumed.

Naturally caffeinated drinks such as coffee and tea are generally safe. The same can't be said for manufactured caffeinated beverages, which don't require FDA approval before distribution. What's more, it is not mandatory for the makers of these drinks to list the exact amount of caffeine on the label. This is cause for concern, because each drink may actually contain up to 400 milligrams of caffeine, which is equivalent to four (8-ounce) cups of coffee. Other undeclared ingredients and proprietary formulas found in manufactured caffeinated beverages may go against the anti-doping codes of many sports organizations. For instance, synephrine is banned by the NCAA, and octopamine is banned by the World Anti-Doping Agency (WADA); both are chemical stimulants found in over-the-counter energy supplements.

moderation. Since one cup of coffee contains 80 to 100 milligrams of caffeine, a maximum of 32 fluid ounces a day is a safe recommendation. Coffee is naturally calorie-free, but if you add sugar, milk, and/or whipped cream, it's an entirely different story. A 16-ounce iced peppermint white chocolate mocha is more like a meal at 500 calories!

MILK

Cow's milk is incredibly nourishing. It helps increase bone mass and build strong teeth, and it also provides nutrients such as calcium, protein, phosphorus, magnesium, vitamin D, potassium, and amino acids. Whenever possible, select 1 percent milk that is organic and grass-fed. Go one step further and choose milk produced by local farmers.

Always go for pasteurized over raw. If you need an alternative to cow's milk, not to worry—there are several:

- Soy milk contains calcium, vitamins B12 and D, and magnesium. It's also high in protein and has all the essential amino acids.
- Almond milk is full of calcium and vitamins D and E, but it is low in protein.
- Cashew milk is rich in calcium and vitamins D and E, but it contains no protein.
- Hemp milk contains calcium, vitamins B12 and D, and riboflavin. It is also high in alpha-linolenic acid but low in protein.
- Coconut milk contains calcium and vitamins A, B12, and D. It doesn't have any protein and is high in saturated fat.
- Rice milk is the least allergenic of all cow's milk alternatives, but it's low in calcium and protein.

Lactose-free milk contains all the wonderful nutrients found in cow's milk but with added enzymes to aid in digestion. Flavored milk may contain all the major nutrients found in unflavored milk, but it also includes sugars, thickeners, emulsifiers, and artificial colors and flavors. Although chocolate milk is advertised as the perfect post-workout beverage, plain cow's milk is just as good for recovery.

Be aware that most dairy-free beverage alternatives have long ingredient lists. Take one glance and you'll see food gum additives, added sugar, and isolated fibers. Unless your purchasing decisions are dictated by medical, religious, or ethical issues, your best bet for your health is to go with milk fresh from the source—the cow. You may also want to consider making your own plant "milk" by blending raw nuts (almonds, cashews, hazelnuts), seeds (hemp, pumpkin, flax), or grains (quinoa, millet, rice, oats) with water. Homemade milks are easy to make, plus they're free of additives and preservatives.

JUICE

Although it's yummy to drink your fruits and veggies, there's no sound evidence that liquid produce is healthier than whole produce. When produce gets "juiced," the end product provides vitamins, minerals, and phytonutrients, similar to that of the whole food, but the fiber is lost in the process. Real juice is free of added sugars, but drinking it is a very easy way to overconsume natural sugars and fat-free calories, compared with eating a whole fruit or vegetable. However, juice is a quick source of fluid, vitamins, and minerals, so athletes might opt for it to assist in rehydration, especially after an intense or long workout or competition, when they lack an appetite for real food. If you want to drink juice after a workout, dilute it with water. Keep to a 1:2 juice-to-water ratio, and add a pinch or two of salt to provide a solution similar to that of a rehydrating sports drink. Also keep in mind that juice uses a different intestinal sugar transporter than glucose. Once in the bloodstream, the beverage is taken up by the liver to be processed into a usable fuel source for the muscles. This can take up to 90 minutes. Because of this, juice isn't recommended as a sports drink during exercise.

ENERGY DRINKS

At one time, energy drinks were synonymous with sports drinks as a way to boost concentration, enhance performance, and delay fatigue. Nowadays, thanks to clever marketing strategies, many people believe that energy drinks, such as 5-Hour Energy, Monster Energy, NOS, Red Bull, and Rockstar, are just as effective as, if not better than, sports drinks. In actuality, most energy drinks contain sugar and calories, while sports drinks are scientifically designed to provide the correct formulation of ingredients to replenish electrolytes, fluids, and carbohydrates.

The purpose of an energy drink is to give you a boost from caffeine and other stimulants. Side effects include dehydration, excessive urination, insomnia, headaches, jitters, restlessness, irritability, and an increased heart rate. If you consume energy drinks in excess, you are at risk of cardiac arrest.

Many athletes rely on energy drinks after a restless night of sleep or during times of high stress and fatigue. Keep in mind that a high-sugar, high-caffeine drink is simply masking your unsustainable lifestyle of being chronically stressed, overtrained, or exhausted. Energy drinks tend to be an abused, addictive, and costly habit. Do yourself a favor and find a healthy alternative to energy drinks, and don't mix them with exercise or alcohol.

ALCOHOL

Some people claim there are health benefits to alcohol consumption, but moderation is key. For healthy adults, moderate alcohol use is defined as one drink a day for women and two drinks a day for men. One drink can be classified as 12 fluid ounces of beer, 5 fluid ounces of wine, or 1½ fluid ounces of distilled spirits.

Heavy drinking is defined as more than three or four drinks a day, or more than eight or 15 drinks a week, for women and men, respectively. As people age, they become more sensitive to alcohol's effects. For men and women 65 years and older, heavy drinking is classified as more than three drinks a day or eight drinks a week.

There are no health benefits to heavy drinking. From an athletic standpoint, the use of alcohol, even in small amounts, can negatively affect hydration status, recovery, sleep, motor skills, motivation, judgment, and overall performance. It can also cause weight gain, nutritional deficiencies, depress immunity, and elevate cortisol (the stress hormone that is linked to weight gain). Because of the large variance of alcohol tolerance among active individuals, athletes are strongly discouraged from consuming alcohol before, during, and after exercise, and during competition season.

FERMENTED FOODS

Before the rise of the food-processing industry, fermented foods and beverages were among the first processed foods consumed by humans. Fermented foods are made with bioactive ingredients and living microorganisms that offer enhanced nutritional and functional properties. Examples include kimchi, sauerkraut, kombucha, tempeh, miso, kefir, and nattō. These products are known to offer great health benefits to an active body.

Fermentation involves using microorganisms such as yeast and bacteria to convert sugar or starches to acid, gas, or alcohol. Let's take a look at one of the mostly popular fermented products available in the grocery store: yogurt. It's essentially the fermentation of lactose by a bacteria that produces lactic acid, which then acts on the milk protein to give yogurt its tart flavor and creamy texture. Fermented foods enhance digestion by providing beneficial bacteria to the gastrointestinal system, which plays a major role in immunoregulation. There's growing research that demonstrates the significant role of fermented and probiotic foods on the human microbiome and immune system. For highly active adults, fermented milk, such as cultured dairy, may improve glucose metabolism and reduce muscle soreness post-exercise. If you are new to fermented foods, start slowly. I recommend consuming only ¼ cup of kefir, kombucha, or sauerkraut a day until you build up a taste tolerance.

Food Intake

Now that you have learned how to properly hydrate, the next step in your nutritional journey is learning how to build a healthy diet. You can't reach your full athletic potential if you aren't providing your body with the nutrients it needs. Each and every meal and snack you consume is an essential part of your training plan.

An optimal diet has many interrelated parts that constantly need adjusting based on your training and competition schedule. For example, calorie and carbohydrate needs are highest on hard training days and right before competitions, to give you long-lasting energy. Protein, high-fiber carbs, and antioxidant-rich foods are important on lighter training days to support health and body composition.

There's a saying in the sports nutrition world: "*You can't out-exercise a poorly planned diet.*" In other words, you must construct a diet that supports the demands of your training. There's no value in putting all of your effort into training but neglecting proper nutrition. While there's no one best diet for everyone, all athletes can learn how to create a solid foundation of eating to support health and fitness aspirations.

EATING APPROACH

Before the food industry turned potatoes into potato chips, chickpeas into hummus, and whole grains into cereals, food was consumed in its real form. It didn't contain chemical preservatives, additives, and artificial flavors, colors, and sweeteners. Unfortunately, with more people feeling overworked, sleep deprived, and constantly on the go these days, convenient, easy, and inexpensive foods are in great demand. Even with an abundance of cookbooks and influential food bloggers, cooking remains too difficult and time-consuming for many people.

Not all processed and fast foods are nutrient-empty. Processed foods such as deli meats and fortified cereals are two examples that come to mind. Health problems occur when chemical processing removes key nutrients and puts in unhealthy additives. Many food sensitivities, diet-related chronic diseases, immune disorders, and gut-related health issues have been linked to the Western diet.

Healthy eating shouldn't be complicated, costly, tasteless, or difficult. In recent years, organic food has grown in popularity, but it's also expensive. If a strict organic diet isn't within your budget, don't worry. Research shows that despite reduced exposure to pesticides and antibiotic-resistant bacteria, organic foods are not nutritionally superior to conventional ones. No single food or food group can provide all the essential nutrients your body needs in one bite, but you can maintain a healthy diet by choosing a variety of foods as close to nature as possible. The more local the food source, the better.

Creating Your Food Plan

Whether you're an elite athlete or a dedicated exerciser, the foundation of any performance-optimizing nutrition plan should do the following:

- Promote good sleep and optimal recovery between sessions
- Support mental, physical, digestive, and hormonal health
- Provide energy and nutrients in sufficient quantities to help you maintain or obtain a healthy body composition and support training demands
- Provide variety, flexibility, enjoyment, and appetite control

To put dietary strategies into action, food guidelines are extremely helpful. Within any diet plan, you'll likely find rules, tips, and strategies to help remove the guesswork and give you confidence in your food-making decisions. The **U.S. Department of**

Agriculture (USDA) has a long history of providing science-based dietary guidance to the American public, but it wasn't until 1992 that the Food Guide Pyramid brought awareness to new food patterns. In 2011, MyPlate was introduced as a new model for eating, complete with a visually engaging way to explain nutrition. However, this style of meal education is limiting for athletes who have specific energy, nutrient, and fluid needs. Moreover, a well-designed training plan that includes high- and low-volume/intensity sessions, rest days, competitions, and an off-season requires nutrition modifications throughout the year. Active individuals must learn to eat in a way that is nutritious and energy-promoting during more rigorous times of training.

Your diet should be personalized just like your training. The next section of this book will teach you how to create a foundation diet: a well-balanced, nutrient-dense style of eating to support your basic energy and nutrient needs. I recommend that you prioritize the following food groups in your meals and snacks:

1. Fruits and vegetables

2. Lean proteins and muscle- and bone-building foods

3. Whole grains and energy-giving carbohydrates

4. Healthy fats

5. Water and hydration-promoting beverages

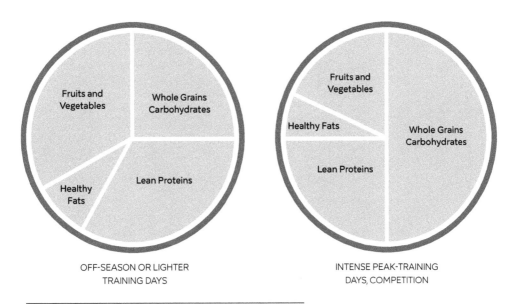

OFF-SEASON OR LIGHTER TRAINING DAYS

INTENSE PEAK-TRAINING DAYS, COMPETITION

Create a performance-enhancing meal in all phases of the season to gain the competitive edge and to protect your health.

Fruits and Vegetables

Role	They fight inflammation, boost immunity, and promote fullness. Great sources of fiber and excellent sources of vitamins and minerals.
Food Examples	Apples, oranges, berries, bananas, mangos, grapes, pineapples, peaches, pears, carrots, beets, broccoli, arugula, spinach, Brussels sprouts, mushrooms
Create Your Plate	Off-season or lighter training days: 40 percent of your meal plate Intense peak-training days, competition: 20 percent of your plate Snacks: One serving per snack
Serving Size Recommendations	1 cup raw or cooked veggies; 2 cups dark leafy greens; 1 cup fruit; 1 whole fruit

TIPS: Add chopped veggies and dark leafy greens to scrambled eggs, then mix that into whole grains and pasta or use it to top a baked potato. Add fruit to oatmeal or other whole-grain porridges, pancakes, and plain yogurt. Once a day, eat a salad, either with a meal or as your meal. Snack on chopped fruits and veggies. Always keep fresh fruits and veggies available. For the most nutrient density, choose local and seasonal produce. Keep frozen veggies on hand. Rinse canned veggies to reduce sodium. If you dislike the taste of raw veggies, serve with hummus, salsa, or smashed avocado. Better yet, grill or bake them to enhance the flavor.

Lean Proteins and Muscle- and Bone-Building Foods

Role	They repair, maintain, and support the growth of muscles and tissues; promote lean muscle mass; build strong bones; provide essential amino acids and iron; and make enzymes and hormones.
Food Examples	Chicken, fish, turkey, sirloin, lean ground beef, pork loin, eggs, cheese, tofu, tempeh, yogurt, edamame, milk or fortified dairy alternatives
Create Your Plate	Off-season or lighter training days: 30 percent of your meal plate Intense peak-training days, competition: 25 percent of your plate Snacks: One serving per snack
Serving Size Recommendations	4 ounces cooked meat; 1 cup milk or milk alternative; 1 cup yogurt; 1 ounce cheese; ½ cup raw firm tofu; 4 ounces raw tempeh

TIPS: Cook proteins in bulk for easy meal prep. Your plate should always contain one serving of a quality protein source. Choose Greek yogurt or cottage cheese to boost protein intake from dairy. Add protein to salads. Look for milk alternatives with at least 6 grams of protein per serving. Choose lean cuts of meat such as skinless white-meat chicken, flank steak, or pork tenderloin. Select nitrate-free processed meats. Keep hardboiled eggs in the refrigerator. Vary your protein throughout the week.

Whole Grains and Energy-Dense Carbohydrates

Role	They are a primary source of energy for the brain and muscles, support high-intensity and prolonged training sessions, and are important for intestinal and heart health. Inadequate intake may increase your risk of injury, illness, burnout, and hormonal issues.
Food Examples	Oats, quinoa, brown rice, barley, bulgur, farro, teff, potatoes, yams, lentils, beans, chickpeas, corn, winter squash, pasta, fresh bread, dried fruits (raisins, dates, figs), honey, syrup
Create Your Plate	Off-season or lighter training days: 25 percent of your meal plate Intense peak-training days, competition: 50 percent of your plate Snacks: One or two servings per snack
Serving Size Recommendations	¾ cup hot cereal; 1 slice fresh bread; 1 cup cooked rice or grain; 1 cup cooked pasta; ½ cup cooked beans or lentils; 1 medium boiled potato (or 1 cup mashed); ¼ cup raisins; 4 pitted dates; ⅓ cup dried figs; 1 tablespoon honey; ⅛ cup syrup

TIPS: Boil or bake potatoes in advance for easy meal prep. Cook a few different whole grains and store in airtight containers in the refrigerator. Replace sweet treats with fruit. Select fresh bread from the bakery instead of processed bread. Make your own granola, muffins, and pancakes. Plant-based sources of protein, such as beans and lentils, and fruits, are also good sources of carbohydrates.

Fluids

Role	They replace water lost through breathing, sweating, and digestion, regulate temperature, promote digestion, maintain body functioning, and reduce fatigue and headaches.
Examples	Plain water, naturally flavored seltzer, mineral water, coffee, tea, milk and milk alternatives (soy milk, almond milk), 100% fruit juice
Create Your Plate	12 to 16 ounces at meals 8 ounces with snacks
Serving Size Recommendations	6 to 8 ounces of coffee or tea; 6 to 8 ounces of milk or juice (Be mindful that milk and juice will add calories to your meal, so prioritize calorie-free plain water.)

TIPS: Add lemon or lime to your water. Set a reminder to drink. Always have a tall glass of water with meals and at snack time. Keep reusable water bottles in the refrigerator for easy consumption. Invest in a filter. Choose naturally flavored sparkling or mineral water instead of regular or diet soda.

Healthy Fats	
Role	They add flavor to meals, slow digestion, promote satiety, store energy, provide insulation, protect organs, absorb nutrients, and provide essential fatty acids.
Food Examples	Canola oil, olive oil, and other plant-based oils; olives, avocados, nut butters, nuts and seeds, fatty fish, chia seeds, hemp seeds, ground flaxseeds, cheese, cream cheese, butter, dark chocolate
Create Your Plate	Off-season or lighter training days: 5 percent of your meal plate Intense peak-training days, competition: 5 percent of your plate Snacks: One serving per snack
Serving Size Recommendations	1 tablespoon oil; 1 tablespoon seeds; 6 ounces cooked fish; 1½ tablespoons nut butter; ¼ avocado; 16 cashews; 45 pistachios; 28 peanuts; 14 walnuts; 23 almonds; 1 tablespoon cream cheese or butter; 1 ounce dark chocolate (70 percent cacao or higher)

TIPS: Portion your fats ahead of time to prevent overindulging. Replace fat-free dairy products (milk, cheese, and yogurt) with 1% fat options. Snack on preportioned unsalted trail mix. Top salads and grains with nuts and seeds. Add butter, oil, and/or cheese to vegetables. Enjoy a piece of dark chocolate at the end of your meal.

Extra Foods	
Role	They bring about enjoyment, add calories and fat, and boost flavors.
Food Examples	Higher-fat meats and dairy, sweetened grains (such as cereal and granola), processed whole grains (such as chips, pretzels, and crackers), desserts Flavor enhancers: herbs, spices, salt, pepper, condiments (such as salsa, mustard, ketchup, Sriracha/hot sauce)
Create Your Plate	Added calories/fat: use sparingly Flavor-enhancers: as needed
Serving Size Recommendations	4 ounces of cooked meat; ½ cup granola; 1 cup cereal; 10 to 15 pretzels, chips, or crackers; ½ cup ice cream; ⅛ teaspoon salt; 1 to 3 teaspoons herbs/spices

TIPS: Extra foods are helpful if you need to gain weight or increase calories around training sessions. Extra foods with higher calories or fat can be included in a well-balanced meal, but it's important to maintain portion control and indulge responsibly.

EATING OUT

People eat out because it's easy and convenient. And dining out is still one of the best ways to celebrate a special occasion or to socialize with friends, family, or coworkers.

About 50 percent of all U.S. food spending is on meals at restaurants and fast-food eateries. Convenience aside, eating out usually means super-size portions that can add calories, sodium, and fat to your diet. It can also be challenging to find a meal that stays within your healthy-eating parameters. Thankfully, many restaurants now cater to the health-conscious eater, and you'll see menus that offer meals with appropriate portion sizes and that contain less sugar and oil—often even made with organic and local ingredients. Some restaurants will even cater to your dietary requests, such as gluten-free or vegan. Because you deserve to eat out on occasion, here are a few tips to make your meal both tasty and good for you:

1. Be inspired to try something new, especially if you are a self-proclaimed picky eater or find yourself stuck in a food rut.

2. Avoid using eating out as a reward or incentive for completing a workout.

3. Review the menu in advance and have an eating plan in place before you arrive at the restaurant. By planning ahead, you'll minimize your chances of overeating. There will be many tempting options, but it's important to consider what you need instead of what you want.

4. Rely on the foundational eating patterns that you have learned in this book to help build a well-balanced meal that will work for your health and performance goals.

Special Diets

Current diet trends include Paleolithic, ketogenic, and Whole30 diets, and intermittent fasting. While you may be looking for a new kind of eating approach to help with your body composition and fitness goals, it's important to note that most special diets are not designed for athletes.

Although religion and culture greatly influence eating habits, the top reasons for restricting specific foods include:

- **Health:** either a diagnosed condition or desired health improvements
- **Body composition changes:** typically a desire for weight loss or decreased fat mass
- **Ethical concerns:** related to animals and/or the environment

Nutrition is a highly recognized component of your athletic performance and health. Following a special diet because you're dissatisfied with your body or in hopes of improving your competitive chances isn't sustainable or practical. A special diet can look attractive when you are slow to achieve your personal goals. However, when that diet becomes extreme and restrictive, there's great risk of declining health, a drop in performance, or even an eating disorder. Your dietary needs depend on your sport type—strength and power, speed, team, or endurance—and your training and personal goals. Most athletes benefit from consultation with a board-certified sports dietitian to navigate the overwhelming number of diets in order to create a safe, maintainable, and health-promoting eating approach for sports success.

VEGETARIAN

An appropriately planned vegetarian diet is a nutritionally adequate way to meet training demands and is suitable for athletes of all levels, from recreational to elite. A vegetarian diet may also reduce the risk of several chronic and lifestyle-related diseases. To promote optimal training, performance, and health, prioritize vegetarian food sources that have essential amino acids, calcium, iron, iodine, magnesium, riboflavin, vitamins B12 and D, and zinc. Due to the high fiber and low energy density of many plant-based foods, athletes may struggle to consume adequate calories on high-volume or high-intensity training days. This can reduce bone density, alter menstrual function, slow metabolism, compromise immunity, and impair physiological functioning. Structuring a vegetarian diet in a way that minimizes excessive fiber consumption around workouts may also reduce the risk of gastrointestinal discomfort. Depending on the type of vegetarianism—lacto, ovo, lacto-ovo, pescatarian (see next page)—some athletes may find it easier or more difficult to adapt this style of eating to different scenarios, such as traveling, eating out, competition schedules, or social events. As with any special diet, athletes will likely need education on the most practical ways to meet energy, macronutrient, vitamin, and mineral needs to support health and fitness goals.

Vegetarian Definition Quick Guide

Types of Vegetarian	Consumes
Vegan	No meat, meat by-products (gelatin, animal broths), animal by-products (eggs, dairy, honey, beeswax)
Lacto-ovo	Dairy, eggs
Ovo	Eggs
Lacto	Dairy
Pescatarian	Fish, seafood, eggs, dairy
Pollotarian	Poultry, fowl, eggs, dairy
Flexitarian	Meat occasionally

VEGAN

Veganism is a style of eating that relies only on plant-based foods. Vegans don't eat any animal products whatsoever. In recent years, several documentaries have showcased the food industry's inhumane practice of factory-farming animals, and athletes with strong ethical beliefs concerning animal welfare may opt for a vegan diet. The Academy of Nutrition and Dietetics states that "appropriately planned vegetarian and vegan diets are healthful, nutritionally adequate and may provide health benefits in the prevention and treatment of certain diseases" and can "meet the needs of competitive athletes."

Performance benefits could include an increased consumption of antioxidants, early satiation from high-fiber foods, and a high carb intake. A vegan diet is also a healthy way to reduce risk of heart disease and cancer. However, poorly constructed vegan diets may predispose athletes to nutrient deficiencies, fatigue, compromised immunity, and increased risk of stress fractures. Because there is not a lot of research about how veganism impacts sports performance, athletes who follow a vegan diet should be monitored regularly by a sports dietitian to ensure that the nutritional demands of their training are being met.

Top Vegan Food Sources

Nutrient	Top Vegan Food Sources
Protein	Tofu, tempeh, soy, grains, beans, lentils
ALA	Flaxseeds, chia seeds, hemp seeds, walnuts
EPA	Seaweed, algae
Vitamin B12	Nutritional yeast, fermented soy, mushrooms, fortified foods, plant milks, supplements
Iron	Legumes, grains, nuts, seeds, fortified foods, blackstrap molasses, dark leafy greens
Zinc	Beans, nuts, oats, wheat germ, nutritional yeast
Calcium	Tofu, fortified foods, plant milks, kale, broccoli, sprouts
Iodine	Seaweed, potatoes, iodized salt
Vitamin D	Supplements

GLUTEN-FREE

Gluten is an amino acid protein, called gliadin, found in wheat. A healthy immune system can identify and neutralize foreign bodies. In autoimmune diseases like celiac, anti-gliadin antibodies attack the body tissue that they would normally protect. As a result, the small intestine villi get damaged, reducing the body's ability to absorb nutrients, so people with celiac disease need to avoid gluten for good. Even the smallest exposure to gluten can set off a cascade of events that negatively affects the immune system and digestive tract.

Gluten-free diets are all the rage right now. I often see athletes going gluten-free as a socially acceptable way to avoid carbohydrates to foster quick weight loss. A gluten-free diet is not necessary or performance-enhancing if you do not have either celiac disease or a gluten intolerance, but there are a few scenarios in which athletes may choose to occasionally experiment with it:

- A temporary avoidance of or reduction in gluten may reduce or minimizes gastrointestinal-related issues during training and competition.
- Individuals who claim to have non-celiac gluten sensitivity may be experiencing FODMAP symptoms (see page 48). These poorly digestible carbohydrates produce symptoms similar to gluten-intolerance.

- When athletes trade bread, beer, and chips for gluten-free whole foods such as fruits, veggies, and whole grains, performance *is* likely to improve, but this is likely the result of eating a more nutritious diet overall, and not necessarily related to it being gluten-free. Heavily processed gluten-free foods, like breads, cereals, bars, and chips, are not healthier just because they're gluten-free.

PALEOLITHIC

Frequently associated with the CrossFit population, the Paleolithic, or Paleo, diet is based on a diet thought to be consumed by our preagricultural, hunter-gatherer ancestors, but has been adapted for today's modern world. The diet claims to be a lifelong pattern of eating that can reduce the risk of chronic disease, control body weight, and improve athletic performance. If you opt to follow a Paleo diet, you must be willing to follow these rules:

Acceptable foods: fresh fruits and vegetables, nuts and seeds (except peanuts), eggs, meats, seafood, grass-fed butter, clarified butter or ghee, coconut oil, cold-pressed plant oils. High-carbohydrate sports nutrition products, like drinks, gels, and bars, are acceptable during longer endurance sessions and immediately after exercise.

Off-limits foods: grains (wheat, rice, corn), dairy products, soy, legumes, salt, processed foods, sugar, artificial ingredients, fast food, and processed meats.

The diet encourages followers to consume 85 percent of their weekly calories within Paleo guidelines. Technically, the diet doesn't have to be low in carbohydrates, but with so many off-limits foods and food groups, including grains, legumes, and dairy, it easily becomes low-carb. Be aware that, as a result, this may compromise training and performance. Even if you eat a healthy Paleo diet, there's still a risk of nutrient deficiencies. Research on the long-term performance effects is inconclusive because most of the literature focuses not on athletes but on adults with comorbidities, such as obesity and type 2 diabetes. The diet can be expensive and time consuming, and it offers little flexibility. On the positive side, it will reduce your consumption of processed and high-sugar foods and increase your intake of whole foods. However, due to the rise in Paleo-approved processed foods, it's debatable whether this is truly a more nutritious lifestyle approach.

KETOGENIC

As mentioned earlier in the book, the ketogenic diet was originally designed in the 1920s for children with epilepsy who didn't respond to medication. Today it has gained popularity as way to quickly induce weight loss in overweight and obese individuals.

The keto diet, as it is commonly referred to, calls for a drastic reduction in carbohydrate consumption, just 20 to 50 grams per day, and for roughly 75 to 80 percent of calories to be consumed from fat. This makes it so the body's glucose reserves are unable to support the central nervous system, so the liver kicks in and forms ketone bodies to act as a source of energy for the muscles and brain. For athletes, the basis of ketosis is to rely less on glucose in order to enhance fat-burning capabilities, thus boosting performance.

Although some research has shown that this low-carb, high-fat diet improves fat oxidation on a cellular level, well-designed research studies on performance under ketosis is lacking. A keto diet can support so-called easy training days, but ketosis itself is physically and mentally limiting during high-intensity and prolonged training sessions, competition, and peak-season training. Side effects include fatigue, low motivation, dizziness, sleep problems, lack of appetite, sickness, injury, digestive issues, and depression.

Despite strong evidence that a ketogenic diet can advance weight loss, there are no guarantees that this diet will help in the long term with weight maintenance, especially when dietary compliance may be challenging. More long-term research is needed before recommending this diet to active individuals.

FODMAPS

FODMAPs is an acronym for fermentable oligosaccharides, disaccharides, monosaccharides, and polyols. They are short-chain oligosaccharide polymers of fructose, galacto-oligosaccharides (**prebiotics**), disaccharides, monosaccharides, and sugar alcohols. In certain individuals, these carbohydrates are poorly absorbed in the small intestine. When they pass into the large intestine, the bacteria located there begins to ferment. This can result in gas, bloating, stomach cramping, abdominal distention, and flatulence. Because gastrointestinal distress is prevalent in athletes and detrimental to their performance, the removal or restriction of FODMAPs may improve symptoms and encourage performance improvements in select individuals suffering from irritable bowel syndrome and gut issues.

Interestingly, when athletes adopt a gluten-free diet to combat gut issues, FODMAPs are likewise decreased and gut-related symptoms often improve. In other words, gluten alone may not be the culprit of the digestive issues that occur in many active individuals. A FODMAP diet can be time-consuming and challenging. Due to its restrictive nature, athletes should consult with a sports dietitian who is experienced with FODMAPs to ensure that dietary elimination is done correctly and safely, and in a way that does not compromise performance and health.

Foods high in FODMAPs include:

- Cauliflower
- Mushrooms
- Apples
- Sorbitol/mannitol/xylitol
- Garlic
- Peas
- Ripe bananas
- Wheat, rye, barley
- Beans and lentils
- Asparagus
- Honey/agave
- Cow, goat, and sheep milk
- Yogurt

INTERMITTENT FASTING

Intermittent fasting involves cycles of alternating eating and fasting. The trend of "not eating" is becoming much more mainstream in our food-obsessed society. This diet isn't so much about what you eat but when you eat. According to this special diet, to optimize health, you should eat sensibly between fasting periods. Binge eating isn't encouraged either. Intermittent fasting strategies include:

- 16-hour fast
- Only eating within an 8-hour window (from noon to 8 p.m.)
- 24-hour fast
- Five days of normal eating with two days a week of only consuming 500 calories (5:2 diet)

During a fasting period, no food is allowed except for water, coffee, tea, and other noncaloric beverages. Fasting appears to have major benefits on insulin resistance. It's been known to reduce blood sugar levels, lower caloric intake, control inflammation, and reduce oxidative stress. Unfortunately, the bulk of research on intermittent fasting and its role in supporting health has been conducted on animals. Much of the research on sports performance in humans has been done on Muslim athletes during the month-long Ramadan fast. It's realistic to assume that sustainable eating practices—outside of religious reasons—are critical to avoid any physical or mental disruptions to training and competition. Hunger is a powerful evolutionary mechanism designed to keep the body fueled and nourished, and you should experience and honor it at least three times a day. More randomized, long-term studies are needed to determine the effectiveness of intermittent fasting on health and weight loss, especially in active individuals. If you are an athlete trying to optimize performance and recovery in your training plan, intermittent fasting is not for you.

PART TWO

Nutrient Timing for Better Results

For several decades, extensive scientific research has focused on nutrient timing: what and when to eat before, during, and immediately after exercise to enhance the adaptive response to exercise. For example, prolonged exercise depletes muscle glycogen storage and breaks down muscle tissue, which increases the risk of fatigue and immunosuppression. Consuming carbohydrates and protein within 30 minutes of working out can help you build muscle, gain energy, and minimize tissue damage. Unfortunately, nutrient timing is a confusing nutrition topic because most strategies conflict with the "healthy" nutrition advice given by experts regarding weight loss and management. For example, a fitness enthusiast may be told to restrict dietary carbohydrates around exercise to lower insulin levels. This can help with fat loss. However, insulin is a powerful anabolic hormone and, with the help of carbs, plays a vital role in transporting amino acids, fatty acids, and glucose from the bloodstream into cells. Although sports nutrition advice may appear "unhealthy," implementing smart fueling practices around and during your workouts is critical for your health and performance. It can reduce the risk of sickness, fatigue, and injury so you can achieve faster results, improving strength, speed, or endurance, while staying consistent with exercise. Read on to learn how you can apply the concept of nutrient timing to your individual exercise regimen.

NUTRIGENOMICS

There's an increasing demand for athletes to use genetic testing to better understand how their DNA influences nutrition and training. Nutrigenomics can show how genes affect the way the human body metabolizes nutrients, and it could help athletes develop a more personalized diet approach to enhance performance while also minimizing health-related setbacks. How does nutrigenomics work? A sports genomic testing company sends you a kit with a specially designed cotton swab that you use to take a DNA sample from the inside of your mouth. You then seal the cotton swab in a protective tube and mail it to a selected DNA lab. Although the tests are not cheap (between $100 and $300) and sports genomics is still in its early phase of development, nutrigenomic testing could be useful in tailoring your nutrition to your body so you can reach your full athletic capabilities.

3

Fueling Before Exercise

If you are a healthy individual and regularly exercise for 30 minutes to 1 hour a day, a well-balanced diet will adequately support your exercise needs. But if your athletic success is dependent on your ability to sustain a repetitive or continuous effort for a physiological adaptation and event readiness, dietary adjustments are necessary to support the training demands placed on your body. The concept of nutrient timing is most important for endurance and ultra-endurance athletes working at maximum aerobic capacity, athletes exercising at threshold levels, and team- or racquet-sport athletes who carry out repetitive high-intensity bursts of activity with variable recovery periods.

Compared with stored energy from fat, the human body has a relatively small storage of carbohydrates (called glycogen) in the body:

- **Muscles:** about 500 grams or 2,000 calories
- **Liver:** about 100 grams or 400 calories
- **Blood glucose:** about 25 grams or 100 calories
- **Adipose tissue (fat):** about 100,000 calories

Carbohydrate storage can deplete within two hours of moderate-intensity exercise. This requires athletes to look for strategic opportunities to ingest carbohydrates to prevent glycogen depletion and support the central nervous system. The next few chapters provide scientific recommendations that will lead to better training and health. The best fueling approach must be personalized to your needs, because the perfect combination of nutrients will be meaningless if I tell you to eat foods that don't interest you, are too expensive, aren't accessible, or give you gastrointestinal issues.

What to Drink Before Exercise

Starting a workout or event in a dehydrated state places you at a competitive disadvantage and poses a health risk. Although strength and short-burst high-intensity athletes are generally less affected by dehydration than endurance and team-sport athletes, it's important for all active individuals to begin exercise in a well-hydrated state. As discussed in chapter 1, even a 2 percent loss in body weight can limit performance. Unfortunately, many athletes chronically go into workouts poorly hydrated. This often results in overdrinking during an athletic event or at the conclusion of the session. Voluntary fluid intake is often insufficient to meet fluid needs. A personalized hydration strategy that accounts for exercise intensity and volume, environment, and personal needs should be part of your training strategy. Well-timed daily and exercise hydration practices will help reduce the risk of dehydration and heat illness, prevent overdrinking, optimize cardiovascular, digestive, and thermoregulatory functioning, enhance recovery, and make for a more enjoyable training session.

What to Drink Before Training

There are many different positions on the best way to achieve appropriate hydration status before physical activity. Although recommendations vary, the overall goal is to ensure that physically active individuals are well-hydrated before exercise. Because sweat rates vary among athletes, customized fluid-intake programs are encouraged.

Pre-workout fluid recommendations:*

- **~4 hours before exercise:** 5 to 7 mL/kg/body weight (bw), or 16 to 20 fluid ounces
- **~1 to 2 hours before exercise:** 3 to 5 mL/kg/bw, or 12 to 16 fluid ounces
- **~10 to 20 minutes before exercise:** 8 to 12 ounces of water

*Adding a small amount of sodium (salt) to a beverage may help stimulate thirst and retain fluids.

How quickly food or drink leaves the stomach is influenced by volume and concentration. Hydrating before exercise will distend the stomach, increasing the ability to optimize the rate at which food and fluid move from your stomach to your small intestine. This rate of gastric emptying occurs rapidly with water but slows down with fluids that contain added calories, carbohydrates, fat, or amino acids. Drinking before a workout doesn't negate your need to continuously drink during the workout; you're still at risk of dehydration and electrolyte disturbances, especially in a hot environment.

Give your bladder sufficient time to empty by timing your fluid intake appropriately with the start of your workout to encourage optimum fluid absorption. In other words, don't wait too late to hydrate. Make sure to drink water before you work out but also remember that consuming too much in a short period can cause excessive urination. Although water should be your first choice, you can also drink milk, coffee, tea, juice, or sports drinks pre-workout. Each type of beverage has benefits and drawbacks, as discussed in chapter 2. Always experiment with what works best for you in different scenarios.

What to Drink Before Competing

Your pre-competition hydration regimen is primarily focused on one goal: for you to begin the competition in a hydrated state. Because dehydration limits your performance, you should start an event "topped off" with fluids. However, you can't store water like a camel does, so once you achieve your full hydration status, any excess fluid will be expelled through urination. And even though urination is a sign of good hydration, urinating too much can cause dehydration. A good general guideline to follow is that if you urinate more than 10 times in a 24-hour period (and your urine is clear), you're probably drinking too much. You may also urinate more often if you're taking high blood pressure medications.

In the days leading up to an event, avoid overdrinking. Respond to your body when you feel thirsty and pay attention to signs of dehydration. If you're participating in a long-distance event during which excessive sweating is likely, you may want to increase sodium in the 48 hours before the event. Add a little sodium (⅛ to ¼ teaspoon) to a 16-ounce bottle of water and consume naturally salty foods, such as pasta sauce, pickles, cottage cheese, pretzels, baked chips, soup, and deli meat. And remember, salty foods stimulate thirst, prompting you to drink. The extra sodium will cause blood plasma volume to expand and may help reduce cardio strain. Because your body tries to dilute extra sodium by holding on to water, you may feel a little bloated.

Recommended pre-competition fluids:

- **Encouraged:** Water, sparkling water, naturally flavored seltzer or mineral water
- **Appropriate:** 100% fruit juices, milk, sports drinks
- **Okay:** Coffee, tea
- **Not recommended:** Energy drinks, alcohol

What to Eat Before Exercise

Consuming carbohydrate-rich foods one to four hours before intermittent, high-intensity, or endurance exercise can help improve performance. Research shows that it helps restore liver glycogen (this is especially true for an early-morning workout), increase muscle glycogen storage, prevent hunger, boost motivation, and it also helps with recovery. Adding protein to a carb-rich pre-workout meal enhances amino acid delivery to the muscles and may attenuate the glycemic response compared with consuming carbohydrates alone. There is a lot of debate over whether athletes should consume carbs before exercise. Let's take a closer look at the most recent chatter on the topic:

- Pre-exercise carb intake in the hour before exercise will impair performance due to reactive hypoglycemia. *Not every athlete is susceptible to this negative reaction, nor does it appear to impact performance after 20 minutes.*
- If carbs are consumed, they should be low on the glycemic index to avoid a rapid drop in blood glucose. *The glycemic index of a pre-workout food doesn't appear to impact performance; choice should be based more on athlete preference.*
- A pre-workout snack of a complex carbohydrate starch, such as the sports drinks UCAN or Vitargo, can blunt the initial spike in serum glucose and insulin to increase fat metabolism. *Slow-absorbing nutrients spend a lot of time in the digestive system, and that may cause gastric distress during intense activity.*
- A high-fat meal will increase fat oxidation and spare muscle glycogen to improve performance. *Despite the metabolic benefits of eating a high-fat meal, in most studies it has not been shown to benefit performance compared with eating a carb-rich meal.*

FASTING

Training in a fasted versus fed state is a popular nutrition intervention to enhance fat burning. Sure, some athletes train on an empty stomach due to lack of time or an aversion to training with food in their stomach. But a good amount of research shows that exercising in a low-carbohydrate or fasted state can induce higher fat oxidation compared with eating before a workout. While training with low carbohydrate storage amounts, also known as "training low," may favor fat metabolism, there's little scientific proof that this leads to enhanced performance on event day. It's also difficult to know if this type of dietary manipulation alone directly assists in weight loss. Lifestyle factors such as overeating, grazing, and inactivity can potentially nullify the fat-burning effects that occur during a fasted training session. While some athletes may experience a favorable change in body composition or a performance boost, not every athlete will respond the same way. Common side effects of training low are fatigue, hunger, sickness, nausea, dehydration, light-headedness, low motivation, and poor recovery. Outside of the lab, it's practical for athletes to work with a sports dietitian to develop a strategic plan for when to consume carbohydrates around workouts to maximize the training responses and meet the demands of competition.

What to Eat Before Training

Athletes exercise at various times during the day and at different intensities and volumes. This makes it difficult to prescribe one standard style of pre-workout eating. And many nutrition prescriptions don't consider the context of the workout or individual goals. Nonetheless, optimal performance requires careful consideration of what, when, and how much you eat before a workout.

MEALS

Digestion is a normal process that takes place when the body is at rest. During exercise, blood diverts away from the gut toward the active muscles and skin. As a result, changes occur in GI motility, blood flow, absorption, and secretions. Consequently, many athletes experience at least one GI symptom, such as bloating, gas, loose stools, or nausea, during exercise. To minimize the potential of upper- or lower-GI distress, carefully make appropriate nutrition choices before a workout. For example, a pre-workout snack of saltine crackers with 2 teaspoons of peanut butter, which has a total of 0.5 grams of fiber, will digest much easier in the hour before exercise than peanut butter on two slices of 100% whole-wheat bread (6 grams fiber). You may need to rely on past experiences and trial and error when fine-tuning your pre-workout meals.

Recommended carbohydrate intake before exercise:

Timing Before Exercise	Carbohydrate	Sample Meal*
1 hour	1g/kg	1 cup cooked rice, 1 cup 1% milk, and 1 cup strawberries
2 hours	2g/kg	1 large potato, ½ cup corn, ½ cup tomato soup, and 2 fig cookie bars
3 hours	3g/kg	1 bagel, 3 slices deli meat or ½ cup tofu, 1 large banana, 1 cup applesauce, 6 ounces yogurt, and 1 cup granola
4 hours	4g/kg	2½ cups cooked pasta, 3 ounces lean meat or tempeh, 2 slices bread, 8 ounces orange juice, 1 small box raisins, 4½ ounces fruit-flavored yogurt, and 1 cup grapes

Examples based on a 150-lb/68-kg individual

When planning your pre-workout meal or snack, remember to:

- Choose foods that are easy to find, prepare, and digest.
- Train your gut by starting with a small quantity, then gradually increasing the amount you consume until tolerable. Allow adequate time to digest food.
- Vary your food choices based on your upcoming workout volume and intensity, weather conditions, and terrain.
- Ingest low- to moderate-glycemic carbs in the 15 minutes before exercise or during the warm-up if you frequently experience a drop in blood sugar (hypoglycemia) at the start of your workout.
- Add a little protein and fat with carbohydrates if you are sensitive to a slight drop in blood glucose.
- Minimize fructose-rich meals because they require time to break down before moving through the blood and into the muscles.
- Minimize high-fat, fiber, and protein foods to prevent feelings of uncomfortable fullness.
- Opt for liquid carbohydrates if you have a sensitive stomach, as they leave the stomach much faster than solids (but be sure not to exceed your recommended fluid intake if only consuming liquid calories).

Carbohydrate consumption leads to a rise in insulin, which increases glucose uptake into muscle cells. Successively, glucose becomes an available fuel source for contracting muscles in the upcoming workout. During this time, however, fat metabolism is suppressed in favor of glucose. For this reason alone, many athletes believe that training in a fasted state will promote better fat burning. However, maintaining the ability to complete high-quality training sessions day after day provides the best scenario to boost fitness and change body composition. Fasting before a workout may interfere with your ability to train long or hard, especially when preparing for a competition.

Here are my top 10 picks for carbohydrate-rich snacks to eat pre-workout (each serving size listed has 25 grams of carbs):

- ¾ cup cooked rice
- ½ cup cooked oatmeal
- 1 English muffin
- 1 slice sourdough bread
- ½ cup applesauce
- 6 ounces yogurt
- 1 small potato
- 10 saltine crackers
- 1 cup grits
- 1 medium banana

These are the top five foods to avoid or minimize because they will put you at risk of intestinal distress:

1. Bulky salads (with dark leafy greens)

2. Foods with bran and high fiber content

3. Broccoli, cabbage, cauliflower, onions, asparagus

4. Sugar alcohols, artificial flavors, sweeteners

5. Beans and lentils

Dietary fiber is the indigestible portion of plant materials that adds bulk to stools and draws water into the intestinal space. It is an important component of a healthy diet, but by temporarily reducing fiber before intense workouts—and in the 24 to 72 hours before a competition—there's less risk of gut issues due to the reduction of residual fiber in the intestinal tract. Bowel movements will still occur, but the goal is to minimize the chances of lower-GI issues such as diarrhea, loose stools, stomach cramping, gas, and bloating.

What to Eat Before Competing

Carbohydrate ingestion before physical activity is designed to spare muscle glycogen, optimize blood glucose levels, boost motivation, delay fatigue, and prevent hunger. Although pre-event nerves can make your appetite disappear, there are clear performance advantages to pre-competition fueling.

Fatigue during prolonged exercise is often, but not always, linked with muscle glycogen depletion and reduced blood glucose concentrations. Eating a carbohydrate-rich meal before a competition can help stave off fatigue. Pre-event foods should be similar to what you'd eat before training. For the "perfect" pre-competition meal, many seasoned athletes rely on rituals and experiences versus science. However, to avoid the potential for GI distress on the one day when you want all your hard work to pay off, you shouldn't deviate too far from scientific nutrition guidelines.

The pre-competition meal should be rich in easy-to-digest carbohydrates and low in fat, protein, and fiber. High-fat foods require lengthy digestion, and carbonated beverages, spicy foods, and certain fruits and veggies (apples and broccoli) may produce gas and bloating. It's not necessary to completely avoid protein, fiber, and fat, though. In small amounts, they help slow digestion, prevent hunger, and stabilize blood sugar levels. Depending on the time of the event, athletes should use nutrition guidelines similar to those for training. As a general rule, allow for:

- 3 to 4 hours to digest a large meal (450 to 800 calories)
- 1½ to 3 hours for a medium-size meal (250 to 450 calories)
- 30 minutes to 1½ hours for a mini meal or snack (100 to 250 calories)

For an early competition, athletes should not forego restful sleep just to eat exactly four hours before competition. It's really what you ate yesterday that fuels your performance for today, and eating three hours prior to the event will allow plenty of time for digestion. If mental and emotional stress mess with your tummy, don't worry. Fuel up well in the 48 hours before competition and eat only as much as you can tolerate on event day. I suggest taking in more liquids than solids.

Get inspiration from this pre-competition meal, designed for a 150-pound athlete to consume three hours before an endurance competition (3g/kg/bw):

- Bagel (48g carbs, 1.5g fat, 4g fiber, 10g protein)
- 1 tablespoon peanut butter (3g carbs, 8g fat, 1g fiber, 4g protein)
- Large banana (31g carbs, 3.5g fiber, 1.5g protein)
- 1 cup nonfat yogurt (47g carbs, 11g protein)
- 3 tablespoons maple syrup (39g carbs)
- 1 cup orange juice (26g carbs, 0.5g fiber, 1.7g protein)
- **Total:** 194g carbs, 9.5g fat, 8.5g fiber, 28g protein

SNACKS

A pre-competition snack isn't necessary if you are still digesting your pre-competition meal. Still, certain scenarios, such as a delayed start, an all-day competition, or an event with heats or periods, may require a snack. The snack may help control hunger pangs, prevent low blood sugar, and top off your fuel tank. Typically, a snack with 30 to 60 grams of carbs and a little protein and fat (5 to 10 grams) is ideal in the 90 minutes before the start of exercise. Your pre-competition snack should be portable and convenient. Choose one of the following:

- 8 to 10 saltine crackers with 1 tablespoon peanut butter
- 1 cup puffed rice cereal with ½ cup yogurt
- 1 rice cake with 1 tablespoon peanut butter and 1 tablespoon honey, and a large banana
- English muffin with 1 tablespoon cream cheese and 2 deli meat slices
- 90- to 120-calorie sports drink
- One packet sports chews
- 100- to 240-calorie sports bar
- 1 ounce hard pretzels with 1 string cheese

Thirty to 50 percent of athletes experience some type of stomach issue before a competition. To avoid this, stick with foods and drinks that are familiar to you.

TIMING OF PRE-COMPETITION MEALS AND SNACKS

Nutrition alone doesn't determine your performance, but it can certainly affect how your body performs in a competitive setting. The key is timing, but it can be difficult to gauge what and when to eat before a competition. Here's a simple strategy for timing your nutrition with your upcoming event.

7 a.m. event: On the day before, eat a large, carb-rich breakfast, a moderate lunch, and a light dinner. On event day, consume your pre-competition meal at 4 a.m.

10 a.m. event: Eat a pre-competition meal at 6 a.m., and a small snack about 90 minutes before the event.

2 p.m. event: Have a small breakfast at 7 a.m. and a pre-competition meal at 10 a.m. If necessary, have a small snack about 90 minutes before the event.

7 p.m. event: Eat a normal breakfast and a light lunch. Snack every 1½ to 2 hours as needed. Have a pre-competition meal three hours before the event.

All-day event: Eat your pre-competition meal about 3 hours before the event starts. Snack on carb-rich pre-workout snacks and fluids throughout the event. Your big meal should wait until the completion of the event.

4

Fueling During and After Exercise

Every sport demands its own physiological and nutritional plan to maximize performance and optimize health. Although fuel and fluid guidelines are easy to prescribe, many athletes struggle to meet individual needs due to performance demands, limited access to drinks and food, lack of appetite, and body composition concerns.

Golf doesn't take a ton of exertion, but it requires timing and precision. Basketball, lacrosse, and ice hockey are intermittent, high-intensity sports requiring strength, power, agility, skill, and aerobic conditioning. In bodybuilding, training and nutrition must be well-matched at all times. Energy expenditure is extremely high in endurance sports such as cycling, cross-country skiing, swimming, and ultra-running. Endurance athletes often struggle to eat and drink enough to meet energy and fluid needs, and it's not uncommon for them to intentionally restrict calories and nutrients due to body-image concerns—a lean body is often considered advantageous for performance. And for high-intensity, short events, such as CrossFit or track and field, diet has less of an impact on performance than do genetics and training.

Regardless of fitness level, every athlete needs a basic understanding of how to fuel and hydrate during and after exercise.

What to Drink During and After Exercise

As you learned earlier in this book, the fluid and sodium needed during exercise vary from person to person. Because sweat rates and fluid intake change throughout the season and vary by athlete and sport, it's impossible to enforce a one-size-fits-all fluid and electrolyte replacement schedule. Some athletes may tolerate a 2 or 3 percent loss of body weight without any effect on performance. On the other hand, athletes who exercise in hot and humid environments, especially at high intensity or for prolonged durations, need to be extra cautious. A hydration strategy must be based on workout intensity, duration, and environmental conditions. The goal is to prevent more than a 2 percent drop in body weight from fluid loss.

A fluid enhanced with sodium can help maintain plasma sodium levels and reduce the risk of overhydration, especially in situations when athletes are likely to overconsume plain water. After exercise, the goal is to fully restore fluid and electrolyte losses before the next exercise session. Sodium consumption from a post-workout beverage promotes fluid retention and stimulates thirst. Recovery is enhanced when protein and carbohydrates are consumed in addition to fluids. For exercise that is high intensity or long duration, or that demands a lot of stops and starts, athletes may experience problems with thermoregulation and fluid loss, especially if the exercise is done at elevated temperatures, in high humidity, or with added clothing and equipment. All of these factors point to the importance of establishing clear hydration goals well before training begins.

What to Drink During Training

Waiting until your brain tells you to drink is a sign that you are slightly dehydrated. It's better for your body to stay one step ahead of your rehydration needs. Sure, not every workout will require a sports drink over plain water, but to promote frequent drinking, make sure you have chilled beverages on hand that are flavorful and palatable.

A well-formulated sports drink should contain the following:

- **Carbohydrates:** 4 to 8 percent solution. To calculate the carbohydrate percentage of a beverage, divide the amount of carbohydrates in one serving (grams) by the amount of fluid in one serving (milliliters) (8 ounces = 240 milliliters). Multiply by 100.
- **Electrolytes:** 0.5 to 0.7 grams of sodium per liter of water, or 250 to 350 milligrams of sodium in 16 ounces of fluid.

Recommended carb intake per hour during exercise*

Type of Activity	Recommended Carb and Electrolyte Intake per Hour	Considerations
Any workout less than 45 minutes, or very low-intensity exercise lasting up to 75 minutes	Not required	Water is recommended. Electrolytes may be necessary for extreme sweat loss. A sports drink "mouth rinse" (swish and spit) may boost reward centers in the brain.
Moderate- to high-intensity exercise lasting up to 75 minutes	Small amounts of carbohydrates from a sports drink	Single or multiple transportable liquid carbohydrates are recommended (i.e., glucose or glucose + fructose).
Endurance or intermittent high-intensity exercise lasting up to 2½ hours	30 to 60g carbohydrates 250mg to 1,000mg sodium 20 to 32oz fluid	Consuming more than 60g of carbs per hour from a single source may cause GI issues. Liquid calories should be prioritized over solids during high-intensity exercise. Sodium provides an osmotic stimulus to retain fluid in the extracellular space. Fructose-only foods (syrup, honey) are not encouraged.
Endurance and ultra-endurance exercise lasting 2½ hours or more	60 to 90g carbohydrates 400mg to 1,000mg or more sodium 20 to 32oz fluid	Multiple carbohydrates (glucose, fructose, maltodextrin) are recommended. Food and/or liquid sources should be palatable. To train the gut to improve gastric emptying and absorption, start with 60 to 70g of carbs per hour.

Carbohydrate-intake recommendations are based on grams per hour, not on body weight.

It's challenging to keep up with fluid intake at appropriate intervals while participating in a strenuous, prolonged, and demanding sports activity. Use training sessions to experiment with different fluid-replacement drinks. Make the effort to identify what products are most tolerable and effective for your competition or regimen. Athletes who lack access to fluids during training, such as trail and road runners, should use hydration packs. Cyclists can rely on bottle cages, while swimmers can keep a bottle on deck.

What to Drink After Training

Unless you take a professional sweat test, it's difficult for you to know precisely how much sodium and fluid you've lost from a workout. However, there are helpful guidelines to follow. To fully restore fluid and electrolyte losses after your workout, aim to consume 24 ounces of fluid for every pound lost. This will help you achieve rapid and total recovery from dehydration. Every pound lost equals about 16 ounces of fluid, so the extra intake should cover obligatory urine losses. Avoid guzzling a large amount of fluid immediately after a workout, though. Instead, drink slowly over a 1-hour period. Drinks should be chilled and slightly flavored to encourage consumption. When your sweat loss is high, try adding at least ¼ teaspoon salt to your beverage (this may not be necessary for all athletes).

Note: Be aware that when you train for long durations, you're also burning fuel that is stored in your muscles and liver. For every gram of stored glycogen, you're also holding on to 3 grams of water. Theoretically, your body weight can drop during exercise without significant loss of total body water. This also explains why many people experience rapid weight loss on a low-carb diet: The immediate weight loss comes from water loss. Thus, weight loss after a hot, prolonged workout may be a combination of glycogen depletion and fluid loss. It's worth it to regularly test your sweat rate during training. This can help you understand how much you're sweating, uncover any symptoms or signs related to dehydration, and determine an action plan to enhance performance without a heat-related setback.

What to Drink During Competition

Better hydration means better performance. It's that simple. Athletes are encouraged to drink early and often, but they shouldn't overdrink. When designing a personalized hydration plan, consider extreme weather or terrain situations, as well as activity intensity. I discourage you from trying anything new on competition day. Instead, test new products and strategies while you're still in training.

Follow these important tips to maintain optimum fluid levels:

- Consume 5 to 8 ounces of fluid every 10 to 15 minutes. One ounce usually equals one gulp. You may need to set a timer to remind yourself to drink during exhausting or high-intensity competitions.
- Choose chilled, slightly sweet (but not overly sweet) beverages.
- Vary the flavors to prevent taste bud fatigue. Complement sweet drinks with savory foods, such as peanut butter pretzel balls (see recipe, page 146) or sour pickles during long-duration, low-intensity exercise.

HOW TO ESTIMATE YOUR SWEAT RATE

Your pre-exercise weight minus your post-exercise weight (in pounds), plus fluid intake (in ounces) during the activity, equals your individual hourly sweat rate. Every 1 pound lost is equal to 16 ounces of fluid. Weigh yourself in the nude. Urination or a bowel movement during the workout will throw off the calculation.

EXAMPLE:

Pre-workout weight: 140 lbs.

Post-workout weight: 139 lbs.

Volume of water consumed during 1-hour workout: 12 oz.

Fluid deficiency (pre-workout weight minus post-workout weight): 140 – 139 = 1 lb. (or 16 oz.)

Total sweat loss: 16 oz. + 12 oz. = 28 oz. per hour

Sweat rate = 28 oz. per hour

- Athletes who participate in sports that require long-distance and high-intensity stamina, such as cross-country skiing, obstacle or adventure racing, off-road running and cycling, endurance or ultra-endurance cycling, open water swimming, or triathlons, should feel comfortable grabbing and drinking fluids on a schedule while moving.
- Reduce your exercise intensity when humidity and temperatures are high to optimize gastric emptying.
- Choose a sports drink over plain water to minimize the risk of hyponatremia, especially if you tend to overdrink water.

What to Drink After Competition

In hot weather, athletes typically desire fluids instead of solid food. Usually, your appetite will wane after an intense competition, when your body temperature is elevated. A smoothie or pre-made recovery beverage is the gold standard of post-competition drinks. Alternatively, athletes competing in the cold will likely choose a hot, often calorie-rich beverage. I encourage you to identify your go-to sources for recovery drinks depending on the demands and environmental conditions of your event.

Regardless of environmental conditions, a liquid protein recovery option consumed within 30 minutes to an hour after a competition will promote muscle tissue repair. However, if you're participating in a sport with fewer than eight hours between events or sessions, prioritize carbohydrates with protein immediately after the first event to kick-start your recovery—otherwise, you'll begin your second event with depleted glycogen stores. The addition of high-quality protein will further enhance recovery between sessions.

If you have no appetite after an intense session, liquid forms of carbohydrate and protein are encouraged. Otherwise, solid food works just fine. A smoothie is a perfect liquid recovery beverage; it is a usually a good source of carbs, protein, electrolytes, and antioxidants, and most people tolerate smoothies well when fatigue, exhaustion, and dehydration linger post-competition.

Here are a few tips to help you choose a healthy post-competition smoothie:

- Review ingredients and nutrition facts to know exactly what you are getting.
- Prioritize protein-based smoothies over all-fruit smoothies.
- Include greens and fruits for extra antioxidants.
- Skip the added sugar, sugar substitutes, juices, and boosters.

If you're making your own smoothie, follow this order of ingredients for the perfect concoction: add liquids, soft foods, powders, and frozen foods to the blender, then the sticky ingredients such as nut butter, honey, or maple syrup.

What to Eat During and After Exercise

By applying scientific nutrition research guidelines to real-world competitive settings, we're seeing more and more athletes excel as never before. Adequate carbohydrate storage is key. When you exercise at moderate intensity, muscle glycogen and blood glucose provide about half of the energy you need, and stored fat provides the rest of it. The higher the workout intensity, the more reliant your body becomes on carbohydrates for fuel. Eating carbohydrates becomes increasingly important during endurance exercise, as the availability of muscle glycogen decreases. The glycogen stored in the liver is only used to maintain blood glucose levels and support the central nervous system. This allows you to continue exercising as long as blood sugar levels are maintained—even in the face of depleted glycogen stores. Proper workout fueling helps you sustain a desirable effort to maximize training adaptations, practice fueling strategies for competition, and protect health. Solid and liquid forms of carbohydrates are equally effective during training, but I encourage athletes to choose the fuel type that is most practical for the duration, intensity, and training demands of a given workout. What you eat after exercising is equally important. Don't forget to consume protein along with carbohydrates. This helps increase net muscle protein balance, promote muscle tissue repair, and synthesize new protein to optimize recovery.

What to Eat During Training

During prolonged or intense training, consuming small amounts of liquid or solid fuel in frequent intervals, before you feel hungry or tired, can help with a host of issues you may encounter while exercising. Ingesting small amounts of fuel every 10 to 15 minutes can prevent an upset stomach, maintain blood glucose levels, promote hydration, and improve central nervous system functioning. Be sure to test any potentially new competition fueling plans during your training sessions, and make every effort to mimic the intensity levels and environmental conditions you will face on event day.

When blood flow to the gut is low because of a redistribution of blood to the working muscles and skin, you should prioritize liquid calories (fluids instead of solids) to promote rapid gastric emptying and intestinal absorption. Scenarios in which this could be an issue include moderate to intense training, training in the heat or engaging in weight-bearing activity. Solid forms of carbohydrates are usually well-tolerated during non–weight-bearing activities, very low intensity endurance activity or cold-weather exercising. In the later scenarios, many athletes enjoy consuming real food along with an electrolyte-rich drink.

Although most nutritional recommendations for training are targeted to endurance athletes, hydration beverages, or sports drinks (see chapter 1), are effective for athletes participating in high-intensity, moderate-duration, or intermittent activities such as CrossFit, soccer, football, basketball, field and ice hockey, swimming, cycling, volleyball, and tennis.

Athletes who participate in extreme sports such as ultra-running, cross-country skiing, and Ironman triathlons have very high carb, electrolyte, and fluid needs to sustain aerobic capacity and meet the metabolic demands of endurance activity. It has been suggested that consuming protein during endurance exercise may offer additional performance benefits compared with only consuming carbohydrates. However, because of conflicting evidence, I don't recommend ingesting protein in a sport drink during endurance exercise.

During the competitive season, training while on a low-carbohydrate diet isn't advised. Training during this time is intense and event-specific, and a low-carb diet can reduce your body's reliance on carbohydrates for fuel, making you a prime candidate for injury, sickness, hormonal disturbances, sleep issues, burnout, and inconsistent training. In the end, this restrictive diet could destroy all of your hard work.

What to Eat After Training

It's well-accepted that a combination of protein and carbohydrates makes the perfect post-workout snack. This pairing helps you achieve the desired training adaptations from your workout by promoting muscle tissue repair and maximizing glycogen synthesis. But does every workout require a protein-packed smoothie? Read on to find out.

MEALS

Specific refueling recommendations depend on a number of issues, among them fitness level, volume and intensity of the workout, body composition goals, menstruation, and daily energy-intake needs. Some athletes prefer a filling meal post-workout, while others desire a lighter snack. What you eat after a workout should contribute to your daily macronutrient and caloric needs. It should also assist in appetite control while keeping your energy levels high throughout the day.

Skip the engineered foods and expensive shakes, and make yourself a healthy, well-balanced meal if:

- You only exercise once a day and have long recovery periods between two workouts.
- Your workout is neither intense nor high volume (i.e., low to moderate intensity for 75 minutes or less).
- You can eat a meal within 45 minutes of the workout.

If the above applies to you, there's no need to go heavy on the carbs and/or protein. Don't worry about the precise amount of macros to eat post-workout. Prioritize real food as much as possible.

Post-workout Meal Options	Carbohydrates	Protein	Fat	Extras (Optional)
Filling meal	½ to ¾ cup oatmeal (measured dry), plus ½ to ¾ cup berries or sliced fresh fruit	1 or 2 hard-boiled eggs, plus 6 to 8 ounces milk of your choice (to add to oatmeal)	2 tablespoons chia seeds or ground flaxseed, plus 2 tablespoons chopped nuts	2 teaspoons each honey and cinnamon
Light meal	2 slices bread or 1 small piece naan; 1 large banana and ½ cup strawberries	¾ cup Greek yogurt	1 to 2 tablespoons nut butter	Drizzle of honey or maple syrup

SNACKS

Certain situations justify having a recovery snack before eating a real meal. I recommend that you eat a snack soon after your workout if:

- There are less than eight hours between two workouts.
- Your workout leaves you completely exhausted (typical of high-intensity, high-volume activity).
- Muscle damage has occurred (typical of plyometrics or weight-bearing activity).
- You are unable to eat a meal within 45 minutes to an hour of your workout.
- Your workout included eccentric movements (downhill running, strength training).

Have a carbohydrate and protein snack within 45 minutes of a workout, when blood flow to your muscles is still high. Then enjoy your real meal whenever you're ready. Because your daily energy and carbohydrate needs are higher on intense or high-volume training days, don't be concerned about the extra calories affecting your body composition goals. Take advantage of this window of opportunity to recover, refuel, and rehydrate to get stronger, faster, and fitter.

The first four hours after a very intense and prolonged workout rank as the best time to achieve your desired training adaptations without compromising your recovery. Your body has just depleted its storage of fuel, muscles are damaged, and your body is very stressed. Consume 1 to 1.2g/kg per hour in the first four hours after exercising. As a simple rule, each hour aim for 50 to 90 grams of carbohydrates and 15 to 25 grams of protein, plus a small amount of fat. Solid or liquid forms of carbs and protein are both acceptable.

Recovery snack suggestions:

- 1 cup milk, ½ cup granola, and 1 cup berries
- 6 oz. plain Greek yogurt, 3 to 4 dates, and ½ to 1 cup cooked rice
- 20g protein powder, 8 oz. milk, and a small muffin or pastry

What to Eat During Competition

Special considerations and attention should be given to fuel and fluids on competition day. Ultimately, what you eat during a competition shouldn't differ drastically from what you eat on training days. Sadly, many athletes tend not to consume enough fuel while training and then overeat on event day for fear of running out of energy. Prior to planning your competition fueling strategy, ask yourself the following questions to help decide if you'll need to consume engineered sports nutrition during your event:

- Are muscle glycogen depletion and hypoglycemia possible during my event?
- Am I at risk of dehydration and a heat illness?

- Will my digestion be compromised by sport intensity or activity?
- Are there unique challenges (i.e., weather, terrain, skills) during the event that will make it difficult for me to meet my energy needs?

If you answered yes to any of the above questions, there are plenty of sports nutrition products available to help you perform your best.

Gels, bars, and chews deliver highly concentrated, portable sources of carbohydrates. The products come in easy-to-open packets or pouches, making them simple to eat during an activity. The flavor, consistency, type, and amount of carbohydrates, as well as electrolyte content, will vary. Popular types of engineered sports nutrition foods include:

BARS

- Amrita nutrition bars
- Base Real Bars
- BumbleBars
- Clif Bars, Clif Kid Zbar, Clif Bar Kit's Organic, and Luna Bars
- EPIC bars
- Gatorade bars
- Hammer Bars
- Health Warrior chia bars
- Honey Stinger energy bars
- KIND bars
- Lara bars
- Odwalla bars
- Picky Bars
- PowerBars
- ProBars
- Raw Revolution bars
- Vega One bars

Tips: Select a bar based on function. Do you want it to fuel your muscles with carbs or to curb your hunger with fat and protein? Look for bars with quality ingredients, that are free of artificial sugars and sweeteners. Ingredients such as rolled oats, dried fruit, and rice are easy-to-digest sources of energy. Proteins, nuts, and seeds will provide satiety but may compromise digestion during high-intensity activities. If you can't find a commercially available sports nutrition bar that meets your needs, you could make your own homemade rice or energy balls (see recipe, page 147), or keep it simple with salty boiled potatoes.

CHEWS AND GELS

- Clif Bloks
- Clif Shots
- E-Gel
- Endura Sports Nutrition gel
- Enervit gel
- Gatorade chews
- Gu chews
- Gu gel
- High5 gel
- Honey Stinger organic chews
- Huma chia energy gel
- PowerBar gel and chews
- ProBar chews
- SIS Go isotonic energy gel
- Sport Beans

Tips: Most gels and chews contain about 100 calories, or 25 grams of carbohydrates, per serving. They're more concentrated in carbohydrates than a sports drink and should be consumed with water to empty them from the gut. For every 25 grams of carbohydrates, drink at least 12 to 16 ounces of water. Some athletes prefer to add the gel to a flask or bottle of water to create a more diluted concentration. Low in sodium (50 to 100 milligrams), gels and chews are ineffective to replenish sodium lost in sweat, but they do provide carbohydrates. Although research shows that carb type (powder, bar, gel) doesn't matter during exercise, it's important to have a well-practiced plan. If you don't, the carbs you ingest will just be sloshing around in your gut, not doing much for your performance.

What to Eat After Competing

A well-designed post-competition nutrition plan plays an important role in replenishing energy storage, repairing damaged muscle tissue, and promoting quick recovery. Many athletes tend to neglect good recovery fueling practices in favor of celebratory foods. From a practical perspective, you should consider post-competition nutrition just as important as post-training nutrition.

MEALS

Immediately after an event, the increased blood flow to your muscles allows for rapid nutrient replacement for growth and maintenance. Back in chapter 1, I talked about how leucine, the branch chain amino acid, is an anabolic trigger—a key activator for muscle protein synthesis and muscle growth. In order for the body to go from a catabolic state, where muscle breaks down, to an anabolic state, where the muscle builds up, it must receive energy from food. Without proper nutrition, catabolism continues to occur, which can destroy muscle tissue. Lucky for you, research tells us that the anabolic window of opportunity is actually open all day. In other words, recovery is everything that happens between two exercise sessions. This is good news because many athletes don't have much of an appetite immediately after competition, and there is no urgency to eat immediately following sports activity. However, muscle cells are more ready to take up glucose and amino acids soon after exercise, so the quicker you can refuel, the better. Glucose and sucrose are twice as effective as fructose in restoring muscle glycogen after exercise. Soft drinks are not recommended as a recovery beverage.

People who participate in triathlons or play a full game of soccer will expend far more energy and lose more fluids than those who engage in low-intensity, precision- and skill-based sports such as golf and curling. A high-carb diet should fully replace muscle glycogen amounts within 24 hours. Athletes who participate in sports that cause extreme muscle damage, like ultra-running, may have impaired muscle glycogen synthesis. Many athletes will experience **delayed onset muscle soreness (DOMS)** for up to 72 hours. Sometimes athletes who forego eating after competition will end up craving foods that are high in fat, calories, and sugar later in the evening, which can compromise recovery and sleep. A post-competition nutrition game plan should take into account the demands of the sport and be designed to help you quickly get back on the field or in the gym.

Post-competition nutrition guidelines include:

- **Less than 2-hour competition:** Consume 1 to 1.2 g/kg/h in the first two hours after competition.
- **2-plus-hour competition:** Consume 1 to 1.2 g/kg/h in the first four hours. As a simple rule, aim for 50 to 90g carbohydrates, plus 15 to 25g protein and a small amount of fat each hour in the first four hours post-event.

For any duration event, prioritize high-quality protein sources and moderate- to high-glycemic carbohydrates, and avoid high-fat foods in the first two hours after competition.

Example of a post-competition meal:

- 4 ounces grilled chicken breast
- Medium baked potato with 1 table-spoon butter
- 1 cup corn
- 1 roll or biscuit
- 12 oz. milk or juice
- ½ cup sherbet
- 1 brownie

SNACKS

Falling short on recovery nutrition places you at risk of illness. That's because intense or endurance competition can suppress the immune system. Although real food is generally encouraged instead of processed food, wholesome foods may not always be practical or feasible immediately after a competition. In many scenarios, a protein powder or meal replacement drink may be useful. If a competition offers a post-event food tent, choose a bagel with cream cheese, chicken wrap, slice of pizza, or milk and pretzels as a snack to assist with recovery. Because your body requires additional energy and nutrients to continue the recovery process, it's recommended that you consume a more substantial meal within two hours after you complete your event.

Short event (less than 1 hour):

    When: Within 30 to 60 minutes post workout (as tolerated)

    What: Recover with a snack. Meal when ready.

    How Much: Snack: 20 to 30g protein and 40 to 60g carbs

    Fluid Intake: 16 to 24 oz.

Moderate-distance event (1 to 3 hours):

    When: Within 30 to 60 minutes post workout (as tolerated)

    What: Recover first with a snack. Meal when ready (within 2 hours post-event)

    How Much: Snack: 25 to 30g protein and 60 to 90g carbs.

    Meal: 20 to 30g protein and 60 to 90g carbs

    Fluid Intake: 16 to 24 oz. in the 60 minutes post-workout. Additional 16 to 24 ounces in the next 90 minutes.

Long-distance event (3 to 10 hours):

    When: Within 30 to 60 minutes post-workout (as tolerated)

    What: Recover first with a snack. Meal when ready (within 2 hours post-event). If possible, eat another meal 3 to 4 hours after the event.

    How Much: Snack: 25 to 30g protein and 60 to 90g carbs.

    Meal #1: 20 to 30g protein and 60 to 90g carbs.

    Meal #2: 20 to 30g protein and 60 to 90g carbs

    Fluid Intake: 16 to 24 ounces every 60 to 90 minutes for the next 4 hours

Recovery snack options:

- 20g whey or vegan protein, 8 oz. milk of your choice, large banana, 1 cup pretzels
- 1 container Greek yogurt, 1 bagel with 1 tbsp. nut butter, and a banana
- 1 cup cooked rice, 12 oz. soy milk, and 1 cup blueberries

5

Fueling on Rest Days

Every athlete and fitness enthusiast will have intentional rest or active recovery days built into his or her training plan. Recovery is crucial because it gives the body time to adapt to the stressors of exercise and heal the mind. Recovery also allows the body to replenish energy storage and repair damaged tissue. On a rest day, it's common for athletes to dramatically cut calories or avoid carbohydrates for fear of gaining weight when energy expenditure is low. Sometimes the opposite occurs, and a rest day is synonymous with a "cheat day." In other words, a rest day is treated as a day to eat foods that are normally off-limits. Improper recovery nutrition may actually hinder your progress and put you at risk of a setback. Consider your rest day a growth day: Use it to fuel and nourish your body so you can become a stronger, fitter, healthier athlete. Remember, sports that include heavy lifting, endurance activity, and all-out efforts can induce excessive inflammation, deplete glycogen storage, and damage tissue and muscles. Your rest day may be the only opportunity you have during the week to strategically consume the right types and quantities of food to maximize recovery between intense training sessions.

What to Drink on Rest Days

Because hydration plays an important role in your health, what you drink on a rest day can help you quickly rehydrate before your next training session so you don't have to worry about exercise-induced dehydration. For protein synthesis to occur efficiently, your muscles must be well hydrated. Without adequate fluid intake, your body won't be able to absorb all the nutrients you consume on your day off because your digestion will be compromised if you're in a dehydrated state. Two of the most common signs of dehydration are fatigue and headaches. Use all of this as motivation to stay on top of your rest-day fluid intake. By doing so, you could find yourself making quicker performance gains with less risk of injury and sickness.

What to Drink on Rest Days Before Training

Every day, you lose water through respiration, evaporation from skin, bowel movements, and your body's metabolic process. Although the exact amount is immeasurable, these insensible water losses can total 1 to 3 liters a day. Consider a day off from exercise a great opportunity to get your body back to a state of optimal fluid balance.

All types of liquid can contribute to your fluid intake, but some are better than others:

Water: This is the best thing to drink for hydration. Aim for at least 12 ounces of water with meals and at snack time. To boost your intake, opt for sparkling water or add a splash of juice, or slices of lime or lemon. Keep a full bottle of cold water with you to remind you to drink.

Milk: Milk contains protein and electrolytes (sodium and potassium). It empties more slowly from your stomach than water does, creating a less dramatic effect on the kidneys. Keep in mind, though, that an 8-ounce serving of 1% cow's milk contains 102 calories, so don't overdo it.

Fruits and vegetables: High-water-content fruits and veggies like watermelon and cucumbers are incredibly refreshing, plus they're rich in fiber, antioxidants, and nutrients.

Caffeinated drinks: Research is mixed on caffeine as a diuretic. However, if you're drinking several cups of coffee in a short time frame, you may get dehydrated from excessive urination.

Sports drinks and juice: Save the money and calories for your more intense and longer training days.

Soda: Plain and simple, soda should not be part of your diet—that includes diet soda—because it contains sugar, artificial flavors, and chemicals, and offers no nutritional value.

Alcohol: If you follow a well-designed recovery nutrition plan, it is probably okay for you to have one alcoholic drink on your day off. But if you drink more than that, you're setting yourself up for delayed recovery. Alcohol elevates cortisol and adds calories to your diet.

What to Drink on Rest Days Before Competing

Coaches often tell athletes that the more they drink, the more they'll pee, and the better they'll perform. It's very common for athletes to drink more fluids than necessary in hopes of arriving to an event in a state of maximum hydration. However, drinking excessively won't solve issues such as cramping, rapid fatigue, headache, or even white salty streaks on clothing. In fact, drinking too much water can be just as harmful as not drinking enough. Consume too much water or diluted sports drinks, and you run the risk of diluting the sodium levels in your blood, which places you at risk of overhydration.

The goal of pre-competition hydration is to deliver you to an event in an optimal state. Aim for 90 to 120 total fluid ounces a day leading up to an event. To ensure a good night of sleep, gradually reduce your fluid intake throughout the evening to avoid unwelcome bathroom trips in the middle of the night. Your urine should have a yellow tint.

As it relates to fluids, balancing sodium levels can be helpful to increasing fluid uptake in the bloodstream. Many athletes eat salty foods or rely on the salt shaker to increase sodium intake; both are practical and affordable ways to optimize sodium levels. Just make sure to drink enough water to balance out the extra sodium: about 16 ounces of water per 1/8 teaspoon of salt. Because sodium acts like a sponge and draws fluids into the extracellular space, some athletes will follow a hyper-hydration protocol to help alter their cardiovascular and thermoregulatory response during exercise. This very simple sodium-loading strategy involves consuming a highly concentrated sodium beverage (1,000 to 1,500 milligrams of sodium) on the night before and morning of a prolonged effort in the heat. Sodium-loading beverages don't just provide sodium, though. Combined with water, they also help expand plasma volume. If you have a history of kidney or blood pressure disorders, always be mindful of your sodium intake.

What to Eat on Rest Days

A proper sports nutrition diet also includes what you eat on nontraining days. Athletes tend to maintain a strict diet on training days, but their rest-day nutrition is often a bit less exact. Knowing what and when to eat on a day when you're expending less energy is easy to do with smart planning. The basis of a training-supportive diet starts with a healthy foundation of eating. What you eat on a day off from exercise should mirror what you would normally eat on a training day. Because your workouts require you to strategically consume slightly more energy from carbohydrates, the major change to your rest-day diet will be the removal of foods and drinks that normally support your training sessions before, during, and after. There's no need to eliminate carbs completely or drastically cut back on calories. Use your rest day as an opportunity to increase your fruit, vegetable, whole-grain, and healthy fat consumption. Go ahead and spend a little extra time in the kitchen preparing meals, but be mindful about grazing and eating mindlessly. If you have a low-intensity, active recovery session in the early morning, say 30 minutes or so, it's okay not to eat before you work out as long as you eat appropriately after the workout.

What to Eat on Rest Days Before Training

A common mistake people make is to restrict food and calories on a rest day. That mind-set is shortsighted. It can take up to 24 hours to fully replenish glycogen storage in the muscles after an intense or long workout, and about 12 hours to restock the liver with fuel. Use your rest day as an opportunity to recover from your previous workouts and fuel up for your next session.

MEALS

Your muscles require fuel and amino acids even when they are resting, so don't skip or skimp on meals on your day off. Focus on food quality instead of quantity; prioritize nutrient-rich foods to optimize health between training sessions. Here are my best-practice tips for rest-day eating:

- Don't intentionally under-eat on a rest day.
- Get the most bang for your buck by eating a variety of wholesome, nutrient-dense foods.
- Have a plan for the day to prevent mindless snacking or overeating.
- Your basic energy needs are, at minimum, 12 to 14 calories per pound of body weight—eating less than this may compromise your hormonal health.
- Carb intake should be 2.25 to 3 grams for every pound of body weight.
- Protein should be 0.8 to 1 gram for every pound of body weight.

While it seems logical that you'd be most hungry on the days when you expend the most energy, it's very normal to feel extra hungry on your days off from training. Experiencing extreme hunger on a day off could be a sign that you are energy deficient—this can happen after a big training day. Or it could be that you're less busy without training and have more time and energy to eat. A voracious appetite could also be a delayed response from previous training. Fluctuations in appetite are completely normal. However, if you have trouble curbing your hunger on rest days, be sure to start the day with a very satisfying breakfast; include fat, protein, and fiber in every meal; and eat a snack every two hours between meals.

Sample rest-day menu:

Breakfast: 2 slices whole-grain bread and a two-egg omelet made with spinach and veggies

Mid-morning snack: Piece of fruit and a small handful nuts

Lunch: Large salad with 1 cup cooked quinoa, 4 ounces protein (fish or tempeh), 1 ounce goat cheese, and a drizzle of olive oil

Mid-afternoon snack: ¾ cup cottage cheese with fresh fruit and 3 dried figs

Dinner: Baked sweet potato with 4 ounces chicken or tofu with 1½ cups steamed veggies drizzled with olive oil

Dessert: Strawberries and 1 ounce dark chocolate

SNACKS

Snacks often have a bad reputation. That's because most people choose ones that are filled with sugar, salt, and artificial ingredients. Choose wisely, though, and snacks will give you the energy you need to survive the day. A smart snack can stabilize your blood sugar, decrease hunger, and fill in nutritional or energy gaps. And if you make the effort to eliminate mindless snacking, you'll reduce unwanted calories. You may have decided to avoid snacks between meals with the goal of losing weight, but going too long without eating can actually slow your metabolism, making weight loss difficult to achieve. That's why it is essential to eat well-timed healthy snacks throughout the day.

Snack ideas:

- 1 string cheese, 10 almonds, and 1 apple
- 6 ounces plain Greek yogurt, a handful of berries, 1 tablespoon chopped nuts or seeds, and a handful of granola
- 4 to 6 dried figs and 1 hardboiled egg
- ½ cup quinoa with 2 tablespoons goat cheese, 1 tablespoon sunflower seeds, and 1 tablespoon raisins, drizzled with olive oil
- 1 pear, 10 to 15 cashews, and 2 slices of deli meat
- 6 to 8 saltine crackers, 1 tablespoon hummus, 1 slice of cheese, and ½ cup edamame in pods
- Apple slices and 20 pistachios

- Veggies and 2 tablespoons hummus (or ½ avocado)
- 6 ounces plain Greek yogurt, handful of fresh berries, and a heaping spoonful of granola
- 1 hardboiled egg, handful of raw broccoli and carrots, and 1 table-spoon hummus

Snack tips:
- Change up your snacks each day based on your appetite, energy, and mood.
- Keep portable snacks on hand (you never know when you'll get stuck in traffic).
- Give your snack purpose: Use it to tide you over until your next meal, fill in nutrient gaps, or control blood sugar.
- Don't go more than 3 or 4 hours without eating.
- Snacks should be like mini meals to help keep you from grazing throughout the day.

What to Eat on Rest Days Before Competing

On a rest day, most athletes worry about eating too much. In contrast, before a competition, they often go to extremes to avoid eating too little. The primary focus of pre-competition eating is to fill the liver and muscles with glycogen to ensure ample energy for the upcoming event. But how much you eat is dependent on the duration, intensity, and timing of your competition.

MEALS

Glycogen is your body's most easily accessible form of energy. Often, athletes load up on carbs to maximize glycogen storage before an event. This is particularly true for events lasting longer than 90 minutes. However, carb loading is about much more than eating a large bowl of pasta on the night before your competition. To completely fill your muscles with glycogen before an endurance event, follow a tapering method. This practice involves drastically reducing training volume 48 to 72 hours prior to a long-distance event and consuming slightly more carbohydrates and less fiber than normal over the course of several meals leading up to the competition. This technique will stock up the storage of glycogen in your muscles and liver, and ultimately help delay fatigue.

Keep in mind that elite or trained athletes store glycogen in greater quantities than novice or untrained athletes. Also, those who normally consume a higher-carb diet will be able to saturate their muscles more effectively with glycogen. To avoid feeling stiff, and heavy, full, and bloated, start your carb loading in the morning, two days out from an event, and slightly reduce your carb intake throughout the day. This strategy works much better than loading up on carbs late in the evening, close to bedtime. To keep from eating every carb in sight, follow this simple carb-loading regimen 36 to 48 hours before an endurance event:

Breakfast: biggest carb meal of the day, with a little protein and fat

Bagel and 3 medium pancakes with maple syrup

Scrambled eggs or turkey sausage

¾ cup yogurt with fruit and chopped nuts

12 ounces orange juice

Lunch: moderate-size meal, low in fiber and fat

Turkey or tofu sandwich on sourdough bread

1 to 2 servings of pretzels or pita chips

Dinner: light meal, minimal fiber and fat

1 to 3 cups rice with 3 to 4 ounces chicken, fish, or tempeh

Bowl of tomato soup

SNACKS

Skipping snacks increases the likelihood of overeating and experiencing hypoglycemia as your day progresses. Make room in your pre-competition diet for energizing snacks. Similar to pre-competition meals, snacks should be low in fiber. Mix and match the following:

- Granola
- Pretzels
- Saltines or rice crackers
- Cereals without whole grains or added fiber or seeds
- Fruit without a peel
- Cooked veggies
- Applesauce
- Yogurt/kefir

Avoid or minimize:

- Gassy veggies like cabbage, broccoli, cauliflower, and Brussels sprouts
- Beans and lentils
- Nuts and seeds
- Fatty meats
- Sugar alcohols/sweeteners

10 healthy pre-competition snacks for the traveling athlete:

1. Fruit leather and jerky
2. Granola bar
3. Pretzels and peanuts
4. Small bagel with nut butter
5. Dried fruit and sweet potato chips
6. Applesauce and powdered peanut butter
7. Granola and shelf-stable milk
8. Tuna packet and saltine crackers
9. Overnight oats
10. Wrap or naan with nut butter and banana

6

Supplements and Performance Enhancers

Although this book takes a food-first approach, it would be a mistake to ignore the many supplements and sports foods marketed to athletes.

Typically, supplements are marketed to athletes and health-seeking individuals to help with weight loss or gain and muscle recovery, to improve immunity and gut health, and for metabolic support. Many athletes look to supplements for a mental or physical edge in training or competition.

It's not uncommon, however, for athletes to use supplements incorrectly—at the wrong time or in the wrong amounts—and then get frustrated because they don't see the promised results.

While not all performance-enhancement supplements are unregulated and unsafe, exceptional marketing strategies and poorly designed research studies can make it difficult to know if a product is truly legit. All athletes, whether novice or elite, need to take responsibility for knowing about the supplements they consume, regardless of recommendations from their coaches or doctors. Sports dietitians are trained to identify sport-specific helpful and harmful supplements. The next section will discuss supplements that athletes commonly use and their impact on athletic performance.

Sports Foods

There is strong evidence for the benefits of consuming sports nutrition products before, during, and after training or competition. Sports foods shouldn't replace real food, though; I recommend that you only use them during sports activities. They provide a palatable and portable source of energy, electrolytes, and fluids to tackle the two main causes of fatigue: dehydration and glycogen depletion. Sports foods are engineered to easily empty from the gut and be quickly absorbed into the small intestine so the working muscles can take hold of the nutrients.

Protein powders such as whey provide an easy method of rapidly repairing damaged tissue after intense training. They can also help boost protein intake among athletes who follow a restrictive diet, such as vegetarians. Leucine, the key amino acid in whey protein, drives the majority of protein synthesis. There's strong evidence that whey protein is a safe and effective recovery supplement. With any sports food, though, you should check all ingredients for safety and effectiveness.

SPORTS DRINKS

Sports drinks are very safe and effective but they're often misused. For a sports drink to work effectively, it should be equal to or less than the osmolality of blood to create a favorable osmotic gradient. Only then can it efficiently deliver fluid, carbohydrates, and electrolytes to the working muscles.

As a reminder, blood plasma has an osmolality of 280 to 300 milliosmoles per kilogram. A sports drink's osmolality is dependent on the particles in a solution. Fluids with an osmolality above 300 milliosmoles per kilogram are considered hypertonic solutions. Isotonic drinks have a similar concentration to that of human blood, about 280 milliosmoles per kilogram. Drinks with a lower osmolality than blood plasma are referred to as hypotonic.

Hypertonic drinks can delay gastric emptying, leaving too much residue lingering in your gut. This sometimes increases the risk of sloshing fluids, bloating, gas, and cramping. It can also cause fluid to shift from working muscles to the gut in an attempt to dilute all the contents in the stomach, increasing the risk of dehydration. This is why both isotonic and hypotonic beverages are encouraged during exercise when a sports drink is advised.

The ideal sports drink should contain sugar (glucose, sucrose, fructose and/or maltodextrin), sodium, potassium, water, and 10 to 14 grams carbohydrates for every 8 ounces. A sodium level of at least 120 milligrams per 8 ounces will enhance the taste to stimulate drinking, facilitate absorption, and maintain body fluids.

The following table lists popular sports drinks and sports drink mixes currently on the market (ranked from lowest to highest sodium content).

Popular Sports Drinks and Sports Drink Mixes

Product	Calories Per Serving	Total Carbs (g)	Sugar (g)	Sodium (mg)	Types of Carb	Extras
Vitargo S2	280	70g	0g	0mg	Fractioned barley amylopectin	Sucralose
CarboPro	200	50g	0g	0mg	Glucose polymers extracted from identity-preserved GMO-free corn	
Hammer Nutrition Heed	100	27g	2g	40mg	Maltodextrin	Xylitol, Stevia
Clif Hydration	40	10g	10g	125mg	Organic glucose, Organic dried cane syrup	
UCAN Sports Drink Mixes	80	20g	0g	130mg	SuperStarch (hydrothermally cooked non-GMO corn)	Xanthan gum, Monk fruit extract
Osmo Hydration (M = male F = female)	35	9g	7g (M) 9g (F)	140mg (M) 184mg (F)	Sucrose, Dextrose	Organic fruit powder
CarboRocket 333	111	27g	7g	142mg	Maltodextrin, Fructose	BCAAs, Caffeinated versions have 50mg caffeine

CONTINUED

Popular Sports Drinks and Sports Drink Mixes

Product	Calories Per Serving	Total Carbs (g)	Sugar (g)	Sodium (mg)	Types of Carb	Extras
NBS Hydration	36	9g	9g	150mg	Organic sucrose, Organic dextrose monohydrate powder	Organic fruit juice powder
Klean Athlete Klean Hydration	60	16g	12g	180mg	Sucrose, Branched cyclic dextrin, Dextrose, Fructose	
Nuun Performance	30	8g	6g	190mg	Dextrose, Cane sugar, Dried fruit powder	
Gatorade Organic Thirst Quencher	120	30g	29g	230mg	Organic cane sugar	
GU Brew	70	18g	9g	250mg	Maltodextrin, Fructose	
Base Hydro	90	21g	Not listed	275mg	Dextrose, Maltodextrin, Fructose	
EFS	96	24g	16g	300mg	Complex carbohydrates, Dextrose, Sucrose	Amino acid blend
Tailwind Nutrition Endurance Fuel	100	25g	25g	303mg	Non-GMO dextrose (glucose), Non-GMO sucrose	Caffeinated version has 35mg caffeine

Popular Sports Drinks and Sports Drink Mixes

Product	Calories Per Serving	Total Carbs (g)	Sugar (g)	Sodium (mg)	Types of Carb	Extras
GU Roctane Ultra Endurance	250	60g	16g	320mg	Maltodex-trin (glucose polymers), Crystalline fructose	BCAAs, Caffeinated versions have 35mg caffeine, Taurine, Beta-alanine
SOS Hydration	10	3g	3g	330mg	Cane sugar, Dextrose	Stevia
CarboRocket Hydration	108	27g	18g	331mg	Maltodextrin, Fructose	Caffeinated version has 35mg caffeine
Skratch Labs Exercise Hydration	80	21g	20g	360mg	Cane sugar, Dextrose	
Infinit Speed	230	57g	21g	379mg	Maltodextrin, Dextrose, Sucrose	
Maurten Drink Mix 160	160	39g	13g	400mg	Maltodextrin, Fructose, Pectin	
EFS-PRO	120	30g	10g	500mg	Long, high-branched amylopec-tin dextrin, Short-chain maltodextrin, Dextrose, Sucrose	Amino acid blend
Precision Hydration 1500	61	15g	15g	750mg	Sugar	

Medical Supplements

Athletes typically use medical supplements because they are experiencing an acute or chronic health issue or a decline in performance, commonly caused by extreme endurance activity, altitude training, and restrictive eating. Having an underlying health issue that impacts nutrient metabolism is another issue. Before using a medical supplement, you should consult with appropriate medical or nutritional personnel, such as a sports dietitian. Here are the most common medical supplements for athletes:

Iron supplements are practical for people with an iron deficiency. Only use if you have **anemia** or iron deficiency, as an excessive intake of iron can be toxic.

Calcium: Dairy sources have the highest bioavailable form of calcium, so I encourage you to opt for them instead of a supplement.

Vitamin D works with calcium to maintain bone health, and is best obtained from sunlight. A blood test is needed to determine proper supplement dosage, which can range from 1,000 to 50,000 IU.

Vitamin B12 is found exclusively in animal products, so vegans may be deficient in it. Though B12 assists in metabolism, exercise doesn't increase your need for it.

Probiotics: Buyer beware, as quality can vary. Choose a probiotic supplement with the right strain or strains for your condition. Probiotics decrease in potency over time, so check the expiration date. The most effective microorganisms are *Lactobacillus* and *Bifidobacterium*. Supplements are costly, so weigh the pros and cons to justify their use.

Performance Supplements

Athletes interested in these types of supplements are generally seeking a direct gain in performance. With so many different types of performance-enhancing supplements on the market, it's difficult for me to provide a universal recommendation. I will discuss two of the most commonly used performance supplements.

The branch chain amino acids (BCAAs)—leucine, isoleucine, and valine—may help endurance athletes delay fatigue. Metabolized in the skeletal muscle, rather than in the liver, BCAAs can be used for energy when glycogen is low and may also help reduce muscle damage, boost mental focus, protect the immune system, and stimulate protein synthesis post-workout. The recommended dosage is 3 to 5 grams pre-, during, or post-workout.

Caffeine is said to enhance fat loss, delay fatigue, and improve focus, attention, and motivation. Because caffeine is absorbed rapidly by the intestinal tract, the optimal time to have it is 45 minutes before performance (~2 to 3 milligrams per kilogram of body weight).

Many supplements are well-supported by research. Examples include **creatine** (increased muscle cell volume and fiber hypertrophy), beet juice (improved skeletal muscle efficiency), and **beta-alanine** (buffer of muscle pH). But this doesn't mean they will work for you. Another example is MCT oil. A triathlete who turns to medium-chain triglyceride (MCT) oil in hopes of a performance boost may end up experiencing diarrhea and an upset stomach, which are common side effects of use. Before purchasing any type of supplement, you must carefully review the research on it. At minimum, choose clean, certified products, and look for the Informed Sport or NSF Certified for Sport seal. Take every initiative to educate yourself on what's in a supplement (and where it comes from), because no supplement is entirely risk-free.

Supplement Polyphenols

Many plant-based chemicals have health benefits. For example, **polyphenols** are micronutrients that naturally occur in plants. They're known to have medicinal properties that can benefit your body. Polyphenols such as quercetin, resveratrol, and curcumin are often touted as having anti-cancer properties, although there is not a lot of research available about their preventive effects on cancer cells. Still, it's natural to assume that a pill or powder form of polyphenols won't be harmful, and that adding them to your supplement regimen will bring health benefits.

Oxidative stress describes an imbalance between free radical production and the body's ability to counteract their harmful effects with antioxidants. Antioxidant supplementation, such as with vitamins C and E, has become a hot topic among athletes as a method to reduce oxidative stress, promote recovery, and enhance performance. However, free radicals serve as important signaling molecules for a number of functions in your body. To get rid of them completely may be counterproductive. The research on whether antioxidant supplementation helps or hinders the adaptive response to exercise, specifically endurance training, is inconclusive. As of now, I can't recommend that you take supplemental forms of antioxidants, but I do encourage you to save your money on pills and instead choose real foods like berries, citrus, and brightly colored vegetables.

Curcumin is another popular supplement touted for its anti-inflammatory and antioxidant properties. It's found in the spice turmeric. Most clinical studies use curcumin extract, not the powder or pill form. More research is needed for me to endorse this supplement as a way to reduce muscle damage and inflammation.

Performance and polyphenol supplements are costly, but because of excessive marketing and glowing testimonials, some athletes are willing to pay for the competitive edge. However, these products may contain undeclared ingredients, contaminants, and banned substances. My suggestion is to use other natural methods to improve your sports performance before turning to these supplements.

Stimulants, Hormone Boosters, Anabolic Steroids, and Prohormones

Doping is the act of using illegal substances to drastically alter the physiology of the human body to improve performance. Unfortunately, in every sport, there's great temptation to use performance-enhancing drugs (PEDs). Anabolic-androgenic steroids are used to improve physical appearance by building muscle. Clenbuterol and ostarine are known to burn fat and build lean muscle mass. Human growth hormone and testosterone, commonly prescribed to older adults to combat age-related decline, can improve muscle protein synthesis. All of these drugs, and many more, are banned by the World Anti-Doping Agency (WADA). It is well-known that body builders, football players, and baseball players have used anabolic steroids to help build muscle and increase body mass. Side effects of such PEDs include aggression, depression, liver damage, cancer, stroke, and blood clots. Among endurance athletes, blood doping with **erythropoietin (EPO)** increases red blood cells to enhance muscle oxygen delivery and delay fatigue. EPO can also thicken the blood, which increases the risk of a heart attack. Whether it's to earn a scholarship, set a personal best, level the playing field, or gain a competitive edge, PEDs aren't a means to an end. There are many other safe and creditable methods to enhance natural talents.

Doping not only threatens the integrity of sports, but it can also compromise health. Resources like Supplement411.org and the WADA website (WADA-AMA.org) can help you identify supplements that violate doping codes. Be sure to check your sport's doping code every year so you know what substances are prohibited in and out of competition.

PART THREE

Optimal Performance for Every Athlete

To create a truly personalized nutrition plan, you need to consider the many factors that impact your food-making decisions. Your age, gender, genetic makeup, stress level, health status, activity routine, body composition, food preferences and restrictions, and socio-economic status all influence the type and quantity of food you consume on a daily basis. As you move through different life stages, your nutritional requirements will change. A growing child needs considerably more calories than a sedentary elderly adult. A new mom can burn up to 640 extra calories a day while producing breast milk, while a post-menopausal woman may struggle to lose weight due to slowed metabolism. Your emotional state also influences what and when you eat. It's completely normal to lose your appetite during a stressful situation, while depression may intensify your appetite. General nutrition guidelines are extremely valuable, but a sports nutrition plan should be tailored to your needs. Since the same dietary advice can't work for everyone, the next chapter focuses on a few important factors to help you better understand your nutrition needs when designing your personal nutrition plan.

7

CHAPTER

Factors Affecting Nutrition Needs

When you embark on designing a sustainable nutrition plan, you'll encounter many challenges, choices, and changes. I like to take a holistic approach. Your diet is not just about eating the "right" foods but also about eating the foods that work for you as a whole person. Your emotions, environment, physical and mental state, and personal values and beliefs will all influence how you eat. Your diet should be well-suited to who you are and what you do, in each stage of your life. Traditional diet plans primarily focus on weight loss and are designed to work for everyone. Chapter 8 will highlight a few gender-specific nutrition considerations that apply to all life stages.

Sex

Men are typically taller, weigh more and have more muscle mass than women. Men also produce large volumes of the hormone **testosterone**, roughly 10 times more than women. This aids in the development and maintenance of lean muscle mass.

Since more calories are needed to sustain lean muscle mass, men naturally have a higher **resting metabolic rate (RMR)** and require more calories. Your RMR is the minimum amount of energy needed to support the body's physiological functions. It accounts for 60 to 75 percent of the total calories your body needs each day. RMR is influenced by your gender, age, weight, diet, and body temperature. Increase your activity level, and you'll see an increased daily caloric expenditure compared with a less active person of the same size, sex, and age.

Women generally have a higher percentage of body fat because of childbearing hormones. Total body fat for women hovers at 25 to 28 percent. This includes essential fat and storage fat. For men, total body fat is 12 to 15 percent. If you regularly participate in sports or exercise, your body may change to meet the demands of the specific activity you do. For example, a healthy female swimmer may have 14 to 24 percent body fat, while a female triathlete may have 10 to 15 percent body fat. Sadly, some athletes practice extreme calorie restriction, taking in far fewer calories than biologically necessary, for reasons related to body-image dissatisfaction and struggles with food. Although men are not immune to health issues, the dieting female athlete is at risk for nutrient deficiencies, hormonal imbalances, eating disorders, menstrual dysfunction, and bone-related issues.

Age

Aging is a natural, often predictable process. Newborns grow amazingly fast and require a lot of nutrients, either from breast milk or formula. Toddlers typically have very strong food likes and dislikes. Food allergies may limit food choices for some children. Tremendous growth and development occur during the teenage years. Due to busy schedules, many young adults rely on heavily processed convenience foods, which increases their risk of being overweight or obese. In adulthood, priorities such as employment and family take time away from self-care and healthy behaviors. About 80 percent of adult Americans live with at least one chronic health condition caused by lifestyle choices.

The mid- to late-life years bring many changes. Weight gain, decreased muscle mass, achy joints, gray hair, and wrinkles are common. But that doesn't mean you can't live an active and healthy life as you grow older. You can use new physical and mental strategies to improve your quality of life and promote graceful aging.

For the elderly, body functions and quality of life can change dramatically. There may be changes in senses of taste and smell, an inability to access healthy food, age-related disabilities and disease, or a lack of a strong social network. Calorie and carbohydrate needs decrease, but fiber intake should stay high to keep the GI tract from becoming sluggish.

In every stage of your life, make proactive choices—consuming nutritious foods and beverages, exercising daily, managing your stress, and refraining from smoking. Taken together, these practices will help improve the quality and length of your life.

Body Composition & Weight

Interestingly, body shape doesn't always indicate whether a person is truly healthy. For example, some people are naturally thin despite being well-fueled and nourished. Others intentionally try to maintain a low body weight through caloric restriction, fasting, and excessive exercise. Understanding the specific composition of your body prior to using diet and/or exercise to change the way you look is the key to weight success without compromising health.

Your body is made up of lean body mass and body fat. **Lean body mass** is the weight of your muscles, bones, ligaments, tendons, and internal organs. Body fat is characterized as either essential fat or storage fat. To fuel movement, fat is stored as triglycerides in the adipose tissue and within the muscle fibers, known as the intramuscular triglycerides. Subcutaneous storage fat is located around the organs and beneath the skin for protection and insulation. An excessive amount of fat, especially around the organs, where it's known as **visceral fat**, increases the risk of chronic health issues such as hypertension, heart disease, and stroke. Essential fat, which is located in the bone marrow, heart, lungs, liver, and muscles, and throughout the central nervous system, is critical for normal body functioning. Given everything that makes up your body, you should understand that a bathroom scale or body mass index chart can't accurately determine your true weight.

Environment

Cold Weather

Athletes don't often associate cold-weather exercise with dehydration, but the condition can happen more easily than you think. First, your thirst response is diminished in the cold, so you may be fooled into thinking that you're properly hydrated because you don't feel thirsty. In cold weather, your body also loses water vapor when you breathe (known as respiratory water loss). Wearing heavy clothing can keep you warm, but this also makes your body expend more energy, which means you sweat more and lose fluids. Finally, when blood is redirected from the extremities to the core, the kidneys aren't told by hormones to conserve water, so urine production increases. It's best to avoid drinking alcohol in cold weather because it dilates blood vessels and contributes to quicker heat loss. Given that the body has to work harder in the cold to maintain homeostasis it makes sense that your appetite for calories—especially a preference for warming food and drinks—is greater during winter months.

Altitude

When the air is thinner, there's less oxygen to breath; the heart beats faster and some body functions, such as digestion, are suppressed. Work capacity is reduced and dehydration risk increases. Because of the loss of appetite, weight loss and a decrease in muscle mass are concerns. Sleep disturbances from episodes of deep and rapid breathing may affect the next day's mood, appetite, and energy levels. It takes 24 to 48 hours for many altitude-related physical symptoms to develop, so an athlete who competes at altitude within 24 hours of arrival may not be affected. It could take two to four weeks for full altitude acclimatization.

8

Considerations for Men and Women

Once upon a time, it was socially unacceptable for women to participate in sports. But in the past few decades, we've seen a rise in women's sports and there are many female athletes with impressive careers. I applaud the gender equality advancement and the major accomplishments made by female athletes, educators, researchers, and coaches. As a female athlete myself, I hope to see more and more women experience the long-term positive effects that athletic activity can bring, including stronger self-image and confidence, and improved mental and physical health. To continue this trend, it's imperative that we consider the unique needs of female athletes. Unfortunately, for a long time, research didn't account for gender differences. Most current nutrition and training recommendations for women still heavily rely on the results of male-focused scientific studies. Considering that men and women differ by 6,500 **genes**, women cannot be viewed as petite men. In this chapter, I will discuss gender nutrition considerations, focusing on a few challenging issues that impact men and women who are pursuing athletic goals.

Considerations for Men

Mental Health

Feelings of never being good enough, extreme thinking, or a perfectionist mind-set could stem from underlying issues of depression, anxiety, addiction, or emotional trauma. Over the years, the issue of depression among elite male athletes has gained national attention. One of the biggest barriers to proper mental health care is stigma. It's not uncommon for male athletes to avoid treating mental health issues because they fear being seen as weak. Male athletes who are extremely concerned about their weight are more likely to suffer from eating disorders and engage in high-risk behaviors such as binge drinking and drug use. Depression or anxiety alongside an eating disorder can exacerbate symptoms and make recovery more difficult. Because athletes are often under a substantial amount of pressure to succeed, I encourage them to carefully balance this pressure with managing their mental health and well-being. Because most mental health illnesses don't improve on their own, it's imperative that you get help when your actions, thoughts, and behaviors frequently cause stress or have an impact on your daily life.

Body Image

Some sports have a history of placing importance on body weight. The mind-set for such sports as gymnastics, horse racing, wrestling, running, ski jumping, rowing, cycling, and triathlon racing is that a low body weight is critical for success. Making matters worse, many coaches applaud athletes who can reduce their body fat to very low levels. Although society tends to place great emphasis on how women look, male athletes aren't exempt from the societal pressures to achieve the perfect athletic physique. An obsessive focus on body fat percentage may lead to unhealthy weight-loss practices, such as starvation; vomiting; the use of laxatives, diet pills, and sauna suits; and excessive exercising—all of which come with long-term health consequences. The goal of any weight-reduction program should be to reduce body fat without compromising health or sports performance. Male athletes who struggle with body image should get professional help—eating disorders are treatable, but they can be fatal without proper treatment.

Considerations for Women

Amenorrhea

Many doctors, coaches, and athletes believe that when women stop getting their period, this is a normal indication of being very fit and active. In reality, menstrual dysfunction is a sign of stress and unhealthy body functioning. Athletic **amenorrhea** isn't merely based on body fat percentage or activity level. Primary causes include energy deficiency, a no- or low-fat diet, severe emotional stress, and intense training. There are two types of amenorrhea:

- **Primary amenorrhea:** regular menstrual periods never started
- **Secondary amenorrhea:** regular menstruation suddenly stops

Amenorrhea may cause stress fractures, loss of lean muscle mass, irreversible bone loss, osteoporosis, and future problems with infertility. Another adverse consequence is an increased risk of cardiovascular disease. It's believed that the loss of estrogen may worsen the function of the **endothelium** (the inner lining of blood vessels), similar to what happens for a post-menopausal woman. The goal of amenorrhea treatment is to increase energy availability by increasing caloric intake and/or decreasing energy expenditure. Although a low-dose oral contraceptive can potentially raise estrogen levels and prevent bone loss, taking supplements or birth control to force menstrual bleeding won't resolve the underlying issue of not eating enough to support exercise demands and normal body functioning.

RED-S

Most athletes train hard to perform at a high level, but you need to acknowledge that your health matters, too. In 2014, the International Olympic Committee (IOC) came up with a comprehensive term, **relative energy deficiency in sport (RED-S)**, to emphasize the wide range of health and performance consequences that occur when energy intake is insufficient to support the energy expenditure required for health. Unlike the **female athlete triad**, a syndrome that includes low energy availability, menstrual dysfunction, and decreased bone mineral density, this newer classification provides a holistic attempt to protect an athlete's psychological and physiological health, while improving performance and longevity in sport. RED-S affects both male and female athletes, and the consequences are numerous: increased injury risk, menstruation dysfunction (for women), impaired judgment, depression, decreased muscle strength, decreased glycogen storage, and diminished performance. Other issues include fatigue, dehydration, low motivation, mood changes, irritability, restless sleep, and disruption to endocrine, cardiovascular, and immunological health.

Menstruation

A regular menstrual cycle is a sign of good health. It's important to understand how a female athlete's hormones may affect performance.

- **Follicular phase (low hormone phase):** Days 1 to 14 of your cycle. For 1 to 7 days, bleeding occurs. Near the end, estrogen levels increase slightly. Strength, power, and high-intensity workouts may be easier to accomplish. Because of menstruation, women require more daily dietary iron than men (18 milligrams a day versus 8 milligrams for men).
- **Luteal phase (high hormone phase):** Days 14 to 28. Progesterone levels increase to prepare the lining of the uterus for egg implantation. Ovulation occurs with a sudden rise in estrogen and luteinizing hormone. If no egg is implanted, progesterone levels drop, the lining sheds, and bleeding occurs to start another monthly cycle. Estrogen may increase fatty acid availability; therefore, low-intensity endurance sessions are recommended because it's easier to utilize fat for fuel. A drop in plasma volume and increase in total body sodium loss could compromise performance in the heat and increase risk of dehydration and hyponatremia.

Every woman responds differently to hormone fluctuations. Common premenstrual symptoms (PMS) include bloating, restless sleep, irritability, and mood swings. You should keep track of your cycle for the purposes of training and competition planning. If you choose to take oral contraceptives to modulate your cycle or prevent pregnancy, discuss the pros and cons with your doctor.

Pregnancy

When a woman is ready to conceive, she should be at her nutritional best. An unhealthy diet and sedentary lifestyle can lead to type 2 diabetes and obesity, and result in difficult labor and birth. To support the growth and development of the fetus, many physiological changes occur in the body. For example, during the first trimester, blood volume and cardiac output increase as various organs require more blood flow. During the second trimester, the mother's heart works 30 to 50 percent harder at rest. Later in your pregnancy, you may experience shortness of breath due to the mechanical alteration of your diaphragm; you will also sweat more. Postpartum, you may struggle to get back to cardio training because you pelvic core is weak. Maternal body fat stored early in pregnancy encourages glucose delivery for fetal needs. A healthy pregnancy weight gain may range from 25 to 40 pounds depending on preconception weight. Not all weight gain during pregnancy is stored as fat. For example, if you deliver a 7.5-pound baby, about 13 pounds of your weight gain is distributed among your breasts, placenta, uterus, blood, amniotic fluid, and maternal fluids. Pregnant women require 27 milligrams of iron and 600 milli-grams of folic acid a day. An exercise prescription should be individually determined for each pregnant woman. Reasons to stop exercise immediately and seek medical advice include:

- Painful uterine contractions
- Bloody vaginal discharge
- Abdominal pain, chest pain
- Sudden swelling or pain
- Blurred vision, headaches, dizziness, faintness
- Extreme fatigue, shortness of breath

Menopause

Menopause is the time in a woman's life when her ovary functioning comes to an end. It typically occurs when a woman is in her 40s or 50s (the average age is 51), and for many women, it can be exhausting and difficult. The perimenopausal transition involves several years of fluctuating hormone levels, particularly a decline in estrogen. Periods become less regular and eventually stop. Common complaints include hot flashes, night sweats, anxiety, depression, concentration problems, vaginal dry-ness, insomnia, headaches, joint and muscle pain, and lower libido. Symptoms differ according to lifestyle, diet, genetics, reproductive history, and culture. Long-term, fluc-tuating hormones may increase the risk of cardiovascular disease, osteoporosis, loss of muscle mass, and weight gain. Medicinal herbs such as black cohosh and dong quai are advertised to help with symptoms, but there is little scientific research to support their safety and effectiveness and warrant usage. Some women look to natural or syn-thetic hormone replacement therapy (HRT) to manage menopausal symptoms, but it's important to consider the risks. A healthy diet along with physical activity, yoga, mas-sage, and meditation are healthy and safe ways to manage the severity of menopausal side effects. Foods such as soybeans, legumes, lentils, tofu and tempeh, flaxseeds, whole grains, beans, and fruits and veggies could reduce some pre- and post-menopausal symptoms because they contain **phytoestrogens**, which are similar in structure to estrogens.

Disordered Eating

It's not uncommon for female athletes to significantly limit caloric intake, believing that a body that weighs less will lead to performance success. Unlike clinical eating disorders, such as anorexia nervosa or bulimia, disordered eating is a general term to describe both harmful eating behaviors used in an attempt to achieve a lower than normal body weight and obsessive behaviors in pursuit of a healthy diet. Examples include rigid or righteous eating, fasting, anxiety, control issues or preoccupation with certain foods, food rituals, extreme concern with body size, and elimination of entire food groups. Body-shaming comments made by coaches and mandatory regular weigh-ins can intensify body image concerns. Because athletes are given a socially acceptable setting in which it's okay to excessively exercise and follow strict eating habits, it's not uncommon for the athletic performance of an energy-starved athlete to be celebrated. But such improvements are regularly short-lived. Eventually, nutrient deficiencies, fatigue, anemia, reduced cardio function, chronic illnesses, injuries, and low motivation will occur and impair physical and mental health. Since disordered eating can be a precursor to a clinical eating disorder, seeking early help is the best preventive measure.

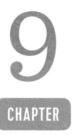

CHAPTER

Considerations for Children and Student Athletes

Nutrition is an important component of sports performance for children and student athletes.

Optimizing daily and sports nutrition enhances athletic performance and reduces the risk of fatigue, injury, or illness, while improving academic ability. By recognizing what foods are best for energy, recovery, and health, and how to time those foods with workouts, young athletes will be able to succeed in all areas of life. While too much food can result in children being overweight or obese, energy shortages can increase their risk of shortened stature, delayed puberty, loss of muscle mass, nutrient deficiencies, and fatigue. One of the most complicated aspects of childhood nutrition is negotiating successful meal planning with a packed school, training, and competition schedule. In addition, picky eating habits, unhealthy food preferences, food insecurity, finances, social networks, and poor sleep can affect sustainable, healthy nutrition practices. Ultimately, kids who eat a healthy and well-balanced diet with appropriately timed meals and snacks will get the nutrients and energy needed to perform well in sports and at school.

Considerations for Children

There are many positive aspects associated with youth participation in sports, such as teamwork, self-confidence, autonomy, and time-management skills. However, sports involvement doesn't offset poorly planned nutrition. Bad eating habits may stop a child or adolescent from achieving adequate growth, development, and health. Although some young athletes are open to changing their eating patterns, many lack an appreciation for healthy food. Nutrition obstacles, such as peer pressure and media influence, a "win at all costs" mind-set, game-day eating, food preferences, and misinformation, can make it difficult for young athletes to meet the demands of their sports and the physiological needs of their developing bodies and minds. Children must recognize that a well-balanced diet will provide nutrients for growth, and that proper sports nutrition can enhance athletic performance by decreasing fatigue and reducing the risk of injury, illness, and dehydration.

A Well-Balanced Diet

An ideal youth diet contains 45 to 65 percent calories from carbohydrates, 10 to 30 percent from protein, and 25 to 35 percent from fat. But children's energy requirements can be as much as 30 percent higher than adults', with energy needs ranging between 44 to 57 calories per kilogram. On the other hand, children who are frequently sedentary need to be carefully monitored. Growth, body mass, and other anthropometric values can determine whether energy intake is adequate. Starting at a very young age, children develop a preference for sweet and nutrient-empty foods and beverages, such as cookies, crackers, chips, candy, and soda. Many of these are high in saturated fats. Educating children about the following nutrients will help them optimize their health, body weight, and performance.

- **Carbohydrates:** Instead of heavily processed foods and calorie-rich beverages, choose whole grains, vegetables, fruits, milk, and yogurt.
- **Protein:** Good protein sources include beef, poultry, fish, eggs, dairy, soy, and legumes.
- **Fat:** Prioritize lean meat, nuts, seeds, low-fat dairy, and olive and canola oils.
- **Important nutrients:**
    1. **Calcium:** Get it from plain yogurt, sardines, mozzarella cheese, low-fat milk, broccoli, cooked spinach, and fortified foods.
    2. **Vitamin D:** Get it from short sun exposure and cow's (or fortified) milk.
    3. **Iron:** Get it from dark leafy greens, fortified whole grains, beans and lentils, and animal protein such as meat, fish, and poultry.

Hydration

Similar to adults, young athletes should carefully monitor and maintain adequate fluid balance to prevent dehydration and heat illness. However, children are at even greater risk of health issues when exercising in hot environments for these reasons:

- Faster metabolic rate
- Greater surface area of skin to lose sweat
- Higher threshold before initiating sweating
- Quick heat absorption
- Reduced ability to dissipate body heat by evaporation

Many young athletes gravitate toward sports drinks, juice, and soda around exercise. Although children athletes can experience detrimental performance effects from dehydration, it's not always necessary to select a sports drink over water. Accounting for sweat rate, sports dynamics, availability of fluids, environmental factors, level of fitness, and duration and intensity of exercise can help determine what beverage is most appropriate around exercise. Fresh fruit, a cold glass of milk, and a handful of pretzels are healthy compromises to a sugary sports drink or soda. Young athletes should start exercise well-hydrated and shouldn't neglect hydration in the 1 to 2 hours post-activity.

Body Weight

Even at a very young age, children and adolescents are concerned about body image. The overweight child may feel intimidated to participate in activities such as dance class, organized sports, or even gym class. In contrast, many young athletes resort to unhealthy weight-control practices, such as skipping meals, vomiting, overexercising, voluntary dehydration, and diet pills. It's not uncommon for five-year-olds to express body dissatisfaction. Most often, kids learn about weight loss from a family member—usually Mom. With age-appropriate education on healthy eating and performance nutrition, young athletes can achieve a weight within a range that is realistic and appropriate to support optimal health, development, and performance.

Game Day

When young athletes participate in multiple games throughout the day, or several events over consecutive days, they often complain of hunger pangs or exhaustion. Just like adults, kids need to optimize performance with smart food choices. To load muscle glycogen storage for the upcoming competition, start the day with a satisfying breakfast, such as oatmeal made with milk and fruit, and a side of yogurt or eggs. For an after-school competition, eat a sustaining lunch. Fatty foods will slow down digestion, leaving you tired and sluggish. Tournaments tend to last all day, often in the heat, so keep hydration and food safety in mind. Foods such as cheese, yogurt, deli meat, and eggs should be stored in a cooler, while granola bars, trail mix, water bottles, and washed fresh fruit can be left in your game-day bag. The body needs 2 to 3 hours to digest a big meal, so keep snacks flowing throughout the day. For the perfect game-day snack, try 15 animal crackers with 1 tablespoon peanut butter and ½ cup unsweetened applesauce.

Considerations for Student Athletes

The student athlete is motivated and driven but still mentally and physically developing. Because of rigorous athletic demands combined with academic pressures and new life responsibilities, it's not uncommon for student athletes to be stressed out and suffer from chronic fatigue, injury, or illness. Many student athletes lack the proper resources to learn about smart nutrition practices that improve sports performance and body composition. The good news is that many high schools and universities now recognize the important roles of the sports dietitian and sports psychologist and provide counseling and educational services to student athletes. Nutrition education is key to better mental and physical health, exercise performance, and the reduced risk of injury and illness. It can also promote better sleep, improve academic performance, and help prevent athletes from using unsafe supplements and performance-enhancing drugs.

Alcohol and Drugs

According to research from the *Journal of Substance Abuse*, individuals involved in athletics are more likely to engage in risky behaviors than non-athletes. Drug and alcohol use can impact recovery, motor skills, strength, power, endurance and sprint performance, and body composition. These substances offer no performance benefits, and student athletes should be educated on the risks of using them (being particularly mindful of binge drinking):

- Hangovers/passing out
- Nausea and vomiting
- Doing something later regretted
- Missing a class or workout
- Doing poorly on a test, assignment, or workout
- Driving under the influence
- Memory loss
- Getting hurt or injured
- Getting in trouble with the police or authorities
- Being taken advantage of (i.e., sexually)

Athletes typically engage in risky behaviors as a way to fit in, suppress uncomfortable or stressful emotions, or induce pleasurable feelings. Student athletes who are serious about their performance need to learn how to avoid the temptation to do drugs or drink alcohol. Never feel embarrassed about saying "no thanks" when drug or alcohol use is encouraged. Friends and teammates who don't respect your choice aren't worth your time—find new people to hang out with who will support your decision to abstain.

Sleep Deprivation

It's not uncommon for student athletes to plow through the school day and training sessions in a sleep-deprived state. A decrease in sleep, particularly from stress, may increase the risk of depression and anxiety. Sleep deprivation can also increase the appetite, intensifying cravings for sugary and fatty foods. Unfortunately, many sleep-deprived student athletes turn to energy drinks to get through the day. The vicious cycle of poor sleep, stress, and unhealthy eating can affect weight, wear down the immune system, and dampen motivation and energy levels. Quality, restful sleep has an enormously positive impact on health and performance. Sleep gives the body a chance to mentally and physically restore itself, helping you feel fresh and alert in the morning. Sleep allows your body to recover from your previous training. Without good sleep, you may notice a decrease in academic and athletic performance. Student athletes should make sleep a top priority. Aim for at least 8 to 9 hours of restful sleep per night, and keep daytime naps to no longer than 30 minutes.

Eating Disorders

Student athletes can be at risk of developing an eating disorder. They usually have high self-expectations and a perfectionist mind-set, and also tend to be involved in sports that overemphasize leanness or body shape. In sports that require a more muscular build, such as soccer, hockey, and cycling, female athletes may struggle with maintaining the necessary fitness level while also wanting to have a "feminine" body. Sometimes the uniform required for a sport can also affect body image. Sports such as diving, swimming, track and field, dance, volleyball, and gymnastics are good examples. Coaches and parents should pay attention to common symptoms of an eating disorder:

- Skipping meals or refusing to eat certain foods or food groups
- Preoccupation with calories
- Extreme mood swings
- Frequent mirror checking for flaws
- Uncomfortable eating around others
- Gastrointestinal complaints (constipation, acid reflux)
- Menstrual irregularities
- Dizziness, light-headedness, fainting
- Sleep problems
- Fine hair
- Dry skin, brittle nails
- Muscle weakness
- Always cold
- Impaired immune functioning
- Feelings of guilt after eating
- Evidence of purging

Eating disorder treatment typically involves a combination of psychological and nutritional counseling. Since there is no one approach that works for everyone, it's important to find the treatment option that works best for each individual.

10

Sport-Specific Nutrition Needs

Different sports require athletes to perform differently depending on intensity, skill, and duration. Nutrition needs vary based on the sport and athlete. For example, soccer, which consists of two 45-minute halves, involves short, intense bursts of activity with occasional rest periods. A player can easily cover more than 5 miles in one game. In contrast, golf is a precision-skill sport requiring focus, concentration, and power to swing the club. Due to misinformation, sports demands, exhaustion, and busy schedules, most athletes fail to meet nutrition guidelines, resulting in performance declines and health issues. Thankfully, sports science and nutrition has advanced over the years to provide easy-to-follow, comprehensive nutrition guidelines.

Endurance and Ultra-Endurance Sports

Preparing for an endurance event requires consistent, year-round training and immense mental focus. Most competitions last anywhere from 90 minutes to 24 hours. Some extend over several consecutive days. Proper nutrition can help delay fatigue, keep motivation high, and reduce risk of injury, sickness, and burnout. The consumption of carbohydrates is vital for endurance and ultra-endurance athletes because carbs keep the brain and nervous system functioning properly, preserve lean muscle mass, and aid in the metabolism of fat. It's not uncommon for endurance athletes to engage in abnormal eating behaviors to achieve a lighter "race weight." Athletes may struggle to meet fuel and fluid requirements during training and competition due to a variety of challenges, including the terrain and weather. Because of the great risk of gastrointestinal distress, I can't overstate the need to practice event-day fueling and hydration strategies while you're training. The off-season is the appropriate time to slowly work toward healthy body composition goals, but it's also a time when athletes may experience unwanted weight gain because they've failed to adjust their energy intake to account for their decreased volume of training.

Ironman Triathlon

An Ironman is a one-day event that has a 17-hour time limit. It involves a 2.4-mile swim, a 112-mile bike ride, and a 26.2-mile run. Elite Ironman athletes typically complete this 140.6-mile distance in 8 to 10 hours. If this is your sport, you must work to maintain a daily energy intake that matches your energy expenditure. Compared with road runners or cyclists, long-distance triathletes aren't greatly penalized for carrying around a little extra body fat. Carbohydrate and energy intake should be regularly adjusted to meet the requirements of each training phase. I highly encourage sports nutrition options such as powders, bars, gels, or chews to meet energy, electrolyte, and fluid requirements during training and competition. Your race-day fueling plan should be built around what you've practiced in training, and based on your individual needs and preferences, weather conditions, and course terrain. Carry sports nutrition products in a variety of flavors and textures to prevent taste bud fatigue. Because rigorous training can decrease the desire to eat, I advise flavorful post-workout high-carbohydrate and high-protein liquid supplements to help meet your energy needs.

Marathon and Trail Running

Typical distances for trail or marathon runners are 26.2 miles, 50 kilometers, 50 miles, and 100 miles. Prior to the event, make sure you know what nutrition will be provided on the course and where the aid stations will be located. Knowing the weather report and the course terrain can also help. Since your gut can't digest nutrition as quickly as you ingest it, you may only be able to tolerate 30 to 60 grams of carbohydrates per hour. A good rule of thumb is to divide your fuel into small doses and consume a dose every 10 to 15 minutes. Because stand-alone runners start an event with fully stocked glycogen storage, this will reduce the risk of bonking (low glycogen or blood sugar) until at least two hours into the event. Use long training sessions to figure out race-day nutrition, including the best products to stave off fatigue. A hydration pack can help with fluid intake. When intensity is low, as in the case of ultra-running, chips, crackers, fruit, pickles, and pretzels can be combined with electrolyte-rich beverages. Avoid high fat and fiber in the 24 to 72 hours before the race to minimize your risk of gastrointestinal issues.

Nordic Skiing

Cross-country skiing is one of the most technically, physically, and mentally demanding sports in the world. It's a full-body workout requiring extreme energy expenditure. In turn, many skiers struggle to consume enough food to compensate, and so on rest days, it is critical for them to eat enough calories to get back into caloric balance. Four to five smaller meals per day should help balance the large energy expenditure that occurs during training. Choose carbohydrates such as fruit juices, muffins, bagels, pastries, cereals/granola, bread, pasta, rice, and potatoes. Dehydration—even in cold temperatures—can reduce blood flow to the muscles. In races lasting more than 80 minutes, it's important to take advantage of the feed zone and replenish with carbohydrates and fluids every 15 to 30 minutes.

Distance Cycling

Preparing for an ultra-distance event, such as a Gran Fondo or a century (100-mile) ride, requires a lot of time in the saddle and a solid nutrition plan. The well-known Race Across America (RAAM) spans 3,000 miles and crosses 12 states. I encourage cyclists to test fueling strategies—including the pre-ride breakfast meal and on-the-go fueling and hydration—multiple times before event day. Cyclists can typically tolerate more calories per hour than runners. However, heavily concentrated carbohydrate solutions (liquid or solid) or overeating at fuel stops could cause abdominal bloating, cramping, and nausea. Instead, nibble on solid food and stay consistent with fluid intake. Chips, pretzels, rice or potato balls, crackers, bananas, cookies, and even small sandwiches are good cycling-friendly foods. Cyclists should consume fuel before they feel hungry or tired. Start fueling within the first 15 minutes on the bike, and continue to fuel every 10 to 15 minutes thereafter to maintain blood glucose levels and optimize hydration.

Open Water Swimming

There's no question that open water swimming is an intimidating sport. Challenges include variable water temperatures, unpredictable water conditions, and unexpected sea life. Except for the 21-mile English Channel swim, marathon swim events are typically 5 kilometers to 10 kilometers. It's easy to forget about hydration while swimming, but swimmers do sweat. Failure to replace fluids and electrolytes can compromise performance. For events lasting more than 90 minutes, consume 6 to 8 ounces of fluid every 10 to 15 minutes, and solid food, such as gels or chews, every 20 to 30 minutes. To avoid losing momentum or getting cold, practice quick stops for food breaks. For cold water conditions, you may prefer hot drinks from a thermos. The optimal fueling strategy is highly personal and involves swimmer preferences and the application of sound nutrition principles.

Strength and Power Sports

Athletes competing in strength and power sports typically have a designated number of opportunities to produce a maximum performance from an explosive single effort. Sometimes, athletes compete in a weight category and may pursue strict dietary restrictions in an effort to "make weight" for competition. Eating disorders, nutrient deficiencies, and distorted body image are pertinent to this unique group of athletes. The primary goal of most strength and power athletes is to build muscle mass. Power athletes spend a lot of time in the weight room to change the physiology of the body to make it more fatigue-resistant. Most of these activities require very short bursts of power. These athletes tend to rely on supplements to help with body composition and performance. But the strategic timing of nutrition to maximize fuel and recovery is the best way to enhance performance while also protecting health.

Bodybuilding

Bodybuilders spend an impressive amount of time perfecting their physique, sometimes up to three hours a day in the gym. It makes sense. After all, their body composition is what they're judged on during competition. The recommended protein intake for bodybuilders is 1.7 to 2 grams per kilogram per day. The tapering phase lasts for about 12 weeks before competition, with the focus on decreasing body fat. If needed, bodybuilders will try to cut more weight through fluid loss to improve muscle definition. The typical bodybuilding diet includes six rigid meals per day. Due to the extreme nature of the sport, bodybuilders can experience distorted body image, muscle dysmorphia, and long-term hormonal and gut issues. Other health risks include immune disturbances, overuse injuries, cardiac issues, and low libido.

Field Events

Field events—high jump, long jump, shot put, and javelin throw—require speed, strength, and power. Skills and body composition will differ, though, depending on the sport. Shot-putters are among the largest athletes on the field and gain mass by weight lifting. High jumpers are usually tall and lean and have a high center of gravity to move the body in the air. They depend on core training, sprint and high jump drills, and plyometrics. Although recommended energy intake varies depending on the individual and the event, typical recommendations are 5 to 7 grams of carbohydrates per kilogram per day and 1.2 to 1.7 grams of protein per kilogram per day.

CrossFit

CrossFit workouts include high-intensity and functional activities such as aerobics, weight lifting, gymnastic movements, and obstacle courses. The diet most frequently associated with CrossFit is the Paleolithic-style diet (Paleo). However, restricting food groups, especially carbohydrates, can prevent athletes from staying consistent with high-intensity workouts. It can also cause fatigue and injuries. Consuming only water during this type of exercise puts individuals at high risk of dehydration and heat illness due to the nature of a typical CrossFit workout.

Rowing

Rowing is a high-energy-expenditure sport that requires great strength, power, and endurance. (Though a standard 2000-meter race lasts 5 to 8 minutes, rowing is still considered a power endurance sport.) Athletes train 4 to 6 hours a day. Rowers compete in either the lightweight or open category. In the open category, there is no defined weight. In the lightweight division, male and female athletes are not permitted to exceed 72.5 kilograms or 59 kilograms, respectively. Often, lightweight rowers voluntarily restrict energy just to make weight. This practice is controversial. After weigh-in, rowers should immediately consume carbohydrate-rich foods and electrolyte drinks to optimize nutrition status before an event. Although some athletes are biologically small and genetically lean, problems can occur with dangerous weight-cutting practices. Dehydration is also a daily concern with rowing because sweat losses can be high. Water bottles should be kept in the coach's boat, at the dock, or with the athlete, to encourage frequent drinking.

Team and Intermittent Sports

Most team sports involve short periods of all-out effort with periods of below-maximum intensities, less-intense efforts, and recovery. To meet sport demands, athletes must train to improve concentration, endurance, strength, and the ability to sprint, jump, or hit on demand. The stop-and-go nature of these sports often results in fatigue as the event continues. As muscle glycogen is depleted, motor skills decline and performance deteriorates. Meeting energy demands is important because glycogen depletion can limit the ability to maintain high-intensity efforts, especially in the later stages of a game. Another major cause of fatigue is dehydration from low fluid intake.

Soccer

Because of the near-constant running that soccer requires, energy expenditure can be high during training and games. Some athletes may play the entire 45 minutes of each half without a substitution. An underfueled player will feel lethargic and have reduced reaction time and speed, and could lose muscle. To help delay fatigue, players are encouraged to consume fluid and carbohydrate/electrolyte drinks early and at regular intervals during games and practices. Because youth soccer players don't sweat as much as adults, the risk of dehydration and heat illness is higher. Soccer players should consume 7 to 10 ounces of fluid every 15 to 20 minutes during training and games. If appetite is suppressed between a tight competition turnaround, a liquid meal replacement beverage may be necessary.

Football

Football involves rapid, high-intensity efforts with short rests between plays. Heavy clothing and excessive sweat losses can lead to serious and potentially life-threatening issues. Body composition varies depending on the position. Receivers are usually lean and fast, while linemen are significantly taller and heavier. Due to the increasing size of football players over the years, there's great concern over physical health. Linemen are three times more likely than the average person to die from cardiovascular disease. Some football players arrive at spring training camps out of shape and overweight, and they turn to quick weight loss methods such as dehydration, appetite suppressants, weight loss pills, severe restrictive calorie diets, and performance-enhancing drugs. Although carbohydrate and protein intake may be high during rigorous training, players need to carefully match energy intake with expenditure to support healthy body composition goals. Long-term health needs should override short-term game-day goals.

Basketball

Basketball requires strength, power, fitness, technical skill, agility, and overall fitness. It's not uncommon for high-profile NBA players to promote extreme diets, from vegan to ketogenic. A restrictive diet isn't necessary for basketball players, though. Athletes should arrive to practices and games adequately fueled and hydrated because glycogen depletion can impair skills and movements. Sipping on fluids throughout practice—during timeouts and at halftime—instead of guzzling them—will optimize hydration status. Basketball players should rehearse game-day eating and hydration strategies during practices. A pre-exercise meal should be low in protein, fiber, and fat. Allow adequate time for digestion. During low-intensity sessions, such as shooting drills, daily carb intake can be slightly reduced.

High- and Very High-Intensity, Short-Duration Sports

The 100-meter hurdle or 50-yard freestyle swimming event are excellent examples of high-intensity, short-duration sports. At very high intensity, maximum efforts will last for less than a minute; at high intensity, effort will last only a few minutes. Training is focused on reaction time, economy, power, skill, mental state, and improving the anaerobic threshold. Since short-duration sports don't substantially reduce muscle glycogen, the breakdown of muscle creatine phosphate (PCr) and the acidosis that occurs from lactate production is typically what limits performance. When athletes are attempting to gain strength or lean muscle mass, strategic timing of nutrition plays a valuable role. Because too much muscle can be just as detrimental as too much body fat, these athletes may struggle with increasing lean mass and improving power while also minimizing body fat to improve speed. In light of this, it's not surprising that performance enhancers and supplements, such as creatine monohydrate, **bicarbonate**, caffeine, and beta-alanine, are often used to increase lean body mass, buffer lactic acid, and improve reaction time.

Gymnastics

The training required to become a successful gymnast is extremely demanding. It involves the repetition of specific skills or individual routines, plus great strength, power, and flexibility. Most gymnasts naturally tend to be short in stature and low in body weight. However, because gymnastics often requires a certain body type, the rates of eating disorders and disordered eating patterns are rather high among gymnasts, often causing delayed menstruation and possibly contributing to stunted growth. It's also no secret that a large number of gymnasts feel pressure—either self-induced or from a coach or judges—to keep their weight as low as possible. This often pushes these young athletes to use diuretics, laxatives, diet pills, and energy drinks for rapid weight loss and maintenance. I never recommend this practice. A diet rich in carbohydrates and protein that includes heart-healthy fats is the ideal. The amount and types of food will vary based on energy needs, training schedule, and body composition goals. If body weight is a concern, I discourage gymnasts from attempting to lose weight during competition season.

Competitive Swimming

Swimming is yet another sport that takes great strength and power, but the typical event is completed in less than 2 minutes. Events and strokes vary in intensity and duration, based on a swimmer's specialty (i.e., sprint, middle distance, or distance). A student athlete swimmer can become chronically fatigued, sleep deprived, and overwhelmed with homework and extracurricular activities. Swimmers require a carb intake of 7 to 12 grams per kilogram per day to compensate for the high energy expenditure demanded by the sport. Best practices include eating a meal in the 2 to 4 hours before competition or an afternoon practice. During a swim meet, swimmers should take advantage of opportunities between events to eat and drink, especially when a meet involves preliminary events and finals. A sports drink is an easy and convenient option. For two-a-day swim practices, it is critical to use a post-workout meal or snack for rapid replenishment of glycogen and fluids and to eat a snack before the early morning session. Due to tight and revealing swimsuits, many female swimmers struggle with body image. It is very important for coaches and athletes to maintain a positive body image atmosphere.

Track Running

Most track events are brief and intense. Athletes may compete several times in one day. While a lean physique may favor the distance runner, track athletes typically have a greater amount of muscle mass in the lower body. During high-volume training, or when an increase in lean muscle mass is desired, you should prioritize a higher energy, carbohydrate, and protein intake, paying special attention to nutrient timing. Track runners may look to supplements to increase muscle mass, buffer lactic acid, and improve reaction time. As discussed earlier, supplements are not without risks. On competition day, they could fail to run to their potential if nerves affect digestion and appetite. Most event concession stands don't provide athlete-friendly foods, so I encourage track runners to pack snacks and drinks for the entire competition day.

Figure Skating

The elegant figure skater needs to have strength and power, endurance and speed, and technique and skill. Highly competitive skaters train twice a day, up to six days per week. I encourage ice skaters to spread food intake over five to six meals a day to help stabilize blood glucose levels, keep metabolism thriving, and reduce hunger and cravings. As in other aesthetic and judged sports, eating disorders remain an ongoing problem. Some skaters feel pressure from coaches and judges to be thin, leading to very restrictive and unhealthy eating practices. I encourage skaters to work with their body instead of fighting it, and to see food as fuel. Not only will proper nutrition improve the quality of figure skating moves, but a healthy diet will also support normal growth and development, and promote longevity in the sport.

11

Nutrition for Weight Loss, Weight Gain, and Weight Maintenance

We all come in different sizes and shapes, based on our unique genetic makeup. However, many of us to turn to exercise to lose weight or gain muscle. Serious athletes are typically more invested in their nutritional needs related to performance—improved endurance, speed, strength, power, and agility. For example, cyclists may want to decrease body fat to improve the power-to-weight ratio, whereas basketball players may attempt to decrease body fat to improve vertical distance. In a contact sport such as football, increased body fat offers a performance advantage. Although athletic success can't be predicted based solely on body weight and composition, both factors may assist in sports enhancements, as long as health isn't compromised. Sports tend to favor specific physiological features, but this doesn't mean you can't excel if you don't have the ideal physique for your sport. The point is, your weight shouldn't be your main focus when you participate in sports. And if you do want to change your weight or body composition, set your goals realistically and your methods accordingly.

Nutrition for Weight Loss

For athletes who have excessive body fat, weight loss may improve health and sports performance. On the other hand, some athletes experience pressure from society, coaches, and judges to lose weight, even if they aren't overweight. When athletes come to me and want to lose weight, the first thing I do is ask why. Then I gather baseline information about their current body composition (in the order listed below) to try to answer the basic question, "What are you made of?"

Determine body composition: There are many reliable body composition assessment techniques to choose from. **Bioelectrical impedance analysis** estimates fat-free body mass through the flow of an electric current. **Dual-energy X-ray absorptiometry (DXA or DEXA)** measures body fat, lean mass, and bone mineral density. **Hydrostatic weighing** is an underwater mechanism that measures body fat percentage. **Air-displacement plethysmography** (Bod Pod) is a whole-body measurement that uses densitometry designed to determine fat versus lean mass. Body composition scales, skin calipers, and handheld devices are popular but not always accurate. Many universities and health centers offer body composition testing at a cost. Urine markers, such as urine-specific gravity and osmolality, can help assess hydration status. Allow at least 2 to 3 months before body composition retesting.

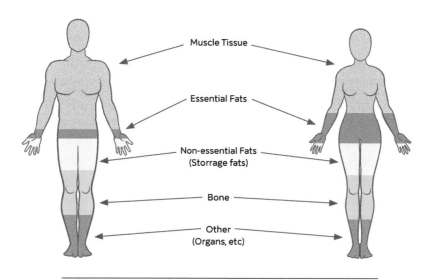

Muscle Tissue

Essential Fats

Non-essential Fats
(Storrage fats)

Bone

Other
(Organs, etc)

Body composition is a measure of muscle, fat, bone and water. Measuring your body composition can give you insight of how much of your body weight comes from muscle and fat.

Determine your target weight: This formula will help you determine your target weight:

Lean weight / (1.0 – desired percentage of body fat)

To maintain hormonal body functioning, body fat should not drop below 5 percent in men and 12 percent in women, or 7 percent in adolescent males and 14 percent in adolescent females. Weight loss should be no more than 0.5 to 1 pound per week. I recommend the Harris-Benedict equation for calculating your total caloric needs, although it won't account for muscle mass. Daily caloric needs of muscular athletes may be underestimated. Don't forget to add your activity factor and use a realistic 2- to 3-month goal weight.

Determine macronutrient needs: Preserving or building lean muscle will require a slightly higher protein intake. Carbohydrate intake should be based on activity and duration. Dietary fats should make up no less than 20 percent of your total caloric needs.

Design a meal plan: A sports dietitian can help you design a personalized performance-focused eating plan to promote gradual weight loss without extreme restrictions, disordered eating behaviors, or use of unsafe products. The best time to change body composition is during the off-season or preparatory phase—outside of competition.

Nutrition for Weight Gain

In a society that's obsessed with weight loss, you may be surprised to hear that some athletes want to get bigger. Extra body fat could benefit athletes such as football and rugby players. In sports that require speed or jumps, increased muscle mass may provide power and vertical height. Self-described "skinny" athletes may find it exhaustingly difficult to gain weight no matter how much they eat. Common reasons for weight-gain struggles are:

- Naturally/genetically slender
- Recovering from an eating disorder
- Underlying medical issue (i.e., overactive thyroid)
- Blunted appetite-regulating hormones
- Lack of accessible food
- Non-sports–related activities (i.e., biking or walking as a mode of transportation)
- Fidgeting

Tips for healthy weight gain:

1. Determine your caloric intake and macronutrient needs based on your weight gain goal (see previous section for formulas). Allow for slow weight gain at a rate of 0.5 to 1 pound every 1 to 2 weeks.

2. Keep a food journal of what, when, and how much you eat.

3. Start by adding 250 to 300 calories to your daily diet. This can come from 20 grams of carbohydrates, 20 grams of protein, and 10 grams of fat. You may experience some digestive distress at first from an increase in calories.

4. Eat frequently throughout the day to prevent uncomfortable fullness. Aim for five to six smaller meals. Eat a well-balanced diet and avoid foods and beverages with little nutritional value, such as chips, candy, and soda.

5. Make every bite count. Choose energy-dense snack foods: granola, homemade energy balls or bars, muffins, dried milk, potatoes, olive oil, avocados, dried fruit, peanut butter, trail mix, pretzels, and yogurt-based drinks.

6. Add extra calories to your dishes in the form of cheese, butter, oil, nuts, and seeds.

7. Change up your diet by incorporating a few liquid meals (or smoothies) each week. Blend in higher-calorie foods such as nut butter, yogurt, and avocado.

8. Never skip breakfast.

9. Focus on good sports nutrition and hydration habits before, during, and after workouts.

10. Carefully design a full-body strength-training program to help build lean muscle mass.

Nutrition for Weight Maintenance

Once you reach your goal weight, the objective is to maintain it. Honestly, this can be extremely challenging for many athletes. Studies show that rebound weight gain happens because of a decline in resting metabolism, the loss of metabolically active tissue, and an increase in hunger. But probably the most common cause is simply neglecting to maintain lifestyle habits that promote long-term weight maintenance. For this reason, I do not recommend extremely restrictive, low-calorie, or rapid-weight-loss diets.

For maximum weight-loss success, make sure your goal weight is appropriate and your nutrition plan does the following:

- Promotes healthy eating habits and optimal health
- Allows for consistent training and optimal sport performance
- Accounts for genetic makeup and family history
- Is age- and height-appropriate
- Encourages normal hormonal functioning
- Does not involve food restrictions, excessive exercise, weight-loss products, or disordered eating behaviors

Many athletes believe that they are at a "healthy," maintainable weight, when, in reality, their body fat or weight is at an unhealthy level—too low. For your safety, the body uses many biological tricks—hormonal, appetite-related, and metabolic—to keep you within a genetically determined "sweet spot" weight range. This is where your body will function at its best, typically within a 5- to 10-pound range. It's important to maintain a realistic weight that works for and not against you; if you try to maintain a weight that is too far below your set point, physiological and psychological issues could occur. The following tips offer practical advice to help you maintain your new weight:

- Make it a lifestyle, not a diet. If your diet requires extreme eating habits, you're likely outside of your healthy weight range. Create healthy habits that you can live with for the rest of your life.
- Be mindful and aware of former unhealthy habits and the times when you feel most tempted to overindulge (i.e., when you're sleep-deprived, stressed, emotional, or hormonal).
- Maintain a high level of activity every day. Even walking has a positive effect on energy expenditure. Choose an exercise routine that you enjoy.
- Change up your exercise routine every 2 to 3 weeks to prevent a plateau. As you get stronger and fitter, gradually increase the intensity.
- Use healthy coping strategies such as meditation or therapy, instead of resorting to food when you feel emotional, stressed, or bored.
- Reduce stress, create a strong support system, and get restful sleep—at least 8 hours a night.
- Weigh yourself weekly and give yourself a healthy weight range fluctuation of 3 to 4 pounds per week. Make small diet and exercise adjustments as needed.
- Learn to love and respect your body at any weight. It's not about how your body looks, but what it can do.

12

Nutrition for Recovery and Immune Function

When an athlete gets sick, it means time away from practice, friends, and school or work. Unfortunately, many athletes (and many people in general) are chronically sick or injured because of academic, financial, physical, and mental stressors. A properly constructed training plan that allows for rest and recovery, coupled with a solid foundational eating plan, can help avoid many illnesses before they start. But if an athlete gets sick, he or she may need to turn to their diet to speed the recovery process. Special considerations should be made during periods of inactivity or rehab for an injury, especially when the athlete is concerned about gaining weight or losing muscle during an extended time away from sports activity. The wonderful thing is that food can be your medicine during periods of compromised health. Each person's immune system is unique, and this chapter will help you better understand the amazing role of nutrition in healing and recovery.

Recovery

Because the body is constantly working to repair and rebuild itself, choosing appropriate foods, with healing nutrients, is key to getting you off the couch and back on the field. While nutrition can't prevent all health issues, there's often a link between an athlete's typical diet and chronic gastrointestinal issues, extreme inflammation, muscle soreness, injuries, and sickness. Building an eating plan with your unique health issues in mind is essential to prevent the onset of a health condition. Plus, the right plan can reduce the longevity of symptoms and get you back in action quickly.

Inflammation

An acute inflammatory response is a normal and necessary adaptation to training. It's also your body's protective response to injury or infection. Sore muscles signal your immune system to repair the small micro-tears that occur in muscle tissue during an intense workout. Some inflammation is beneficial, but an excess can damage cells and increase free radical production and oxidative stress, impairing adaptations to exercise. This is why training programs should allow you to slowly adapt to exercise fluctuations (in distance, intensity, and skill) to reduce excessive inflammation. But injuries are different. It isn't until inflammation subsides that the body can begin to recover from trauma.

To reduce pain and muscle soreness, or to accelerate return to play after an injury, athletes frequently rely on **nonsteroidal anti-inflammatory drugs (NSAIDs)** such as ibuprofen (Advil) and naproxen (Aleve). However, these drugs aren't without side effects. Overuse can cause a delay in musculoskeletal tissue repair and bone healing. NSAIDs can also damage your digestive tract and kidneys. If NSAIDs are prescribed, make sure to use the lowest dose possible, for the shortest time possible. Nutrition plays a key role in promoting and combating the inflammatory process. Instead of a pill, look to your plate to help reduce inflammation.

- **Omega-3 fatty acids:** salmon, herring, chia seeds, walnuts, canola oil, flaxseed oil
- **Vitamin C:** guava, pineapples, red and green peppers, kiwi, oranges, strawberries
- **Vitamin E:** almonds, Swiss chard, spinach, turnip greens, kale, plant oils
- **Polyphenols:** celery, onions, ginger, garlic, chocolate, coffee, tea, olive oil, apples, berries
- **Prebiotics:** legumes, berries, Jerusalem artichokes, asparagus, garlic, leeks
- **Probiotics:** sauerkraut, kimchi, kombucha, kefir, tempeh, miso

Gastrointestinal (GI) Issues

GI issues frequently impair performance and recovery. This can come in the form of an upset stomach, vomiting, or diarrhea. GI symptoms are often caused by reduced blood flow to the gut, especially when you jump or bounce. For example, during running, blood flow to the digestive system is impaired, so the stomach may reject ingested food or fluids, sending them out of the body—either up or down. Common upper- and lower-GI issues are outlined in the following table.

Upper-GI Issues	Lower-GI Issues
Nausea	Intestinal cramping
Vomiting	Side stitch
Stomach pain/cramps	Gas
Bloating	Loose stools/diarrhea
Belching	Intestinal bleeding
Heartburn/reflux	Urgency to defecate

The severity of GI issues depends on the athlete and sport. The high-impact nature of running may jostle the gastric system, contributing to diarrhea. In cycling, posture on the bike may increase pressure on the abdomen, causing stomach pain, acid reflux, and cramping. For swimmers, swallowing air from short and rapid breathing can cause belching. Additionally, using a straw-based hydration system or gulping fluids, especially carbonated drinks, may cause **aerophagia**, which is excessive and repetitive swallowing of air, and belching. To reduce the risk of GI issues during exercise, follow these practical guidelines:

- Avoid NSAIDs, especially on competition day. They're associated with an increased risk of GI complications, mucosal bleeding, and ulcers.
- If you're lactose-intolerant, replace dairy with a lactose- or dairy-free alternative on high-intensity training or competition days.
- In the 4 to 24 hours before an intense or long-duration activity, minimize or avoid high-fiber foods such as cruciferous veggies and fiber-rich cereals or grains. Choose potatoes and plain breads instead.
- Avoid high-fructose beverages and foods such as soda, juice, and candy, as well as carbonated drinks, around workouts and competition.
- Stay well hydrated.

- Allow 4 to 6 weeks to train your gut to improve intestinal absorption with ingested foods and fluids.
- Use trial and error before and during training or competition to figure out what foods work and don't work for your gut.

Injury

Whether you are a highly trained athlete or a fitness enthusiast, there's always a risk of injury. Bruises and cuts are minor injuries, while an ACL tear, rotator cuff impingement, stress fracture, or ruptured Achilles tendon are classified as serious injuries.

Nutrition is vital in the healing and rehab process for every type of injury. Along with the right type of retraining program, smart dietary habits can help athletes come back after an injury sometimes even stronger and faster than before. Because the injured body has altered nutrient and energy needs, the following recommendations can help expedite your return to sports activity:

- **Protein:** While the precise amount varies, be sure to keep up with your protein intake, especially after exercise or rehabilitation to maintain strength and muscle mass. Aim for 1.5 to 1.8 grams per kilogram per day.
- **Carbohydrates:** Slightly lower your normal carbohydrate intake to prevent excessive weight gain. Focus on consuming high-fiber and whole-grain foods, along with fruits and veggies.
- **Fat:** Prioritize plant and fish oils to decrease inflammation, but be mindful of portion sizes.
- **Vitamins and minerals:** Calcium, zinc, and vitamins A, C, and D all aid in wound healing, immune function, tissue repair, and cell growth. For bone health, consume three servings a day of foods and beverages that are rich in calcium and vitamin D. This is not only dairy, but also nondairy fortified items such as orange juice and soy milk.
- **Hydration:** To help deliver nutrients and support your joints and soft tissue, stay well hydrated with 90 to 120 ounces of fluid per day.
- **Calories:** Some athletes feel that they should limit calories and/or carbs when they're not expending calories. But your body still requires energy and nutrients, even at rest. And if you've had surgery, your daily energy needs could increase by 10 to 20 percent. For most athletes, a 5- to 7-pound weight gain is nothing to be concerned about. Once you return to your sport, you'll quickly shed that weight.

Muscle Soreness

Most athletes are familiar with delayed onset muscle soreness (DOMS). This is the pain and stiffness felt in the muscles after strenuous or unaccustomed exercise. DOMS is frequently associated with high-force eccentric contractions, such as running downhill, CrossFit routines, or weight training. DOMS typically lasts between 24 and 72 hours, but you may not feel the soreness start until two days after exercise—hence the word "delayed." Sometimes DOMS is so severe that you may feel injured. There is no clear explanation for why DOMS occurs, but I recommend skipping the NSAIDs and trying these interventions instead:

Tart cherry juice: For an extra boost on top of whole-food antioxidants, consume 4 to 8 ounces of tart cherry juice before and/or immediately after you exercise. It can help reduce inflammation and help with muscle recovery. After extreme exercise, drink the juice once a day for the following 48 hours.

Coffee: Consumed before exercise, caffeine may help reduce the perception of pain and soreness during exercise. Consumed in the days after strenuous resistance training, it may also reduce the onset of DOMS. The recommended intake of caffeine is 3 milligrams per kilogram of body weight in the 45 minutes before exercise, and up to three cups of coffee per day.

Non-nutrition methods: Outside of the kitchen, Epsom salt baths, light foam rolling, recovery boots, massage and non–weight-bearing cardio can help reduce inflammation. Ice is another option to reduce inflammation. However, research shows that cold water immersion (ice bath) and **cryotherapy** (cold chambers) are no more effective for reducing inflammation after workout or competition than recovery methods like riding a bicycle or active stretching.

Immune Function

Exercise has positive and negative effects on the immune system. Moderate daily activity may enhance the immune system. In contrast, excessive amounts of prolonged, high-intensity exercise can have a temporary depressive effect on immune function. This explains why so many athletes get sick in the week or two following a competition. Normally, your body does an exceptional job of recognizing and fighting against foreign invaders. But psychological stress, physical exhaustion, restless sleep, environmental stress, travel, and/or inadequate nutrition can take a toll on your immune system, placing you at greater risk of infection or illness. Much of your immune system exists in your GI tract, so it's worth exploring nutritional strategies to help you boost your immunity to support your extremely active lifestyle.

Gut Health

The health of your gastrointestinal system is extremely important to your immunity. There are about 100 trillion live microorganisms in your gut. They work to promote normal GI function, protect the body from infection, eliminate invading pathogens, maintain healthy tissue, and regulate metabolism. Interestingly, about 75 percent of your immune system is in the gut. There's a growing scientific interest in the relationship between gut health, mood, and metabolism. New research suggests that the microbiota in your gut may play a larger role in your body's adaptive process to exercise than originally thought. Various factors, such as what you eat, how you exercise, and your environment and genetics, influence your internal bacteria. Remember, a healthy gut means a healthy body and mind, so pay close attention to your daily needs and make good lifestyle choices for a happy tummy.

Antibiotics

Antibiotics are medications that help save lives. They fight off very harmful bacteria. However, it's widely believed that antibiotics are overprescribed in the United States. The concern is that these medications can't distinguish between good bacteria and bad bacteria and end up destroying everything in their path. Antibiotics can alter the normal bacteria in your gut and weaken your intestinal microbiome. Some people advocate the use of collagen or bone broth to heal the gut lining and reduce intestinal inflammation, but there's not enough research on this practice for me to recommend it. Instead, repopulate the healthy gut bacteria by following a whole-food, nutrient-dense diet and choosing probiotic foods that are fermented. If you are taking an antibiotic, scale back your training until you finish your entire course of treatment and increase consumption of probiotic-rich foods. If your doctor gives you permission to exercise, start slowly and monitor your body for side effects. Be on the lookout for shortness of breath, rash, yeast infection, diarrhea, abdominal cramps, and/or vomiting.

Lifestyle Factors

Your immunity doesn't depend on a single factor. A host of lifestyle factors—including sleep patterns, stress management, and exercise regimen—influence your immune system. When one gets out of whack—for instance, if you have a restless night of sleep—your immune system will feel the disruption right away. Although many supplemental teas and products claim to boost or support immunity, your first line of defense should be real food. To keep your immune system healthy and strong, adopt these lifelong healthy-living strategies:

- Participate in daily exercise
- Don't smoke
- Maintain a healthy weight
- Get restful sleep
- Drink alcohol in moderation (if you choose to drink)
- Eat a diet rich in fruits and vegetables
- Partake in good hygiene practices (i.e., regular handwashing)
- Practice food safety
- Maintain health and nutrition practices when you travel
- Practice stress management
- Drink clean water

Chronic Health Issues

Learning that you have a chronic health condition can be frightening, confusing, and life-changing. In addition to the normal everyday challenges you face, chronic illness adds a new level of stress, isolation, and discomfort, not to mention financial pressures. It's true that a chronic illness diagnosis affects your life and long-term goals, but a healthy diet and exercise regimen can help you manage symptoms, build confidence, and develop adaptability. Pain, fatigue, and debilitating symptoms can keep you on an emotional rollercoaster, so I encourage you to focus on aspects of your life that you can control, including your mind-set. Above all, don't ever stop believing in yourself and your athletic dreams—no matter how long it takes you to get there. In spite of your illness, you can find a healthy way to continue to live the life you want to live.

Allergies

Allergies can occur at any age. Sometimes they disappear for a few years, then come back. When you have an allergy, your immune system makes **antibodies** that identify a particular allergen as harmful. When you come into contact with that allergen, your immune system reacts by inflaming your skin, sinuses, airway, or digestive system. Reactions can be mild to severe, and in some cases, such as anaphylaxis, life-threatening.

Common allergy types ar

- Food
- Skin
- Dust
- Insect sting
- Pollen
- Pets
- Drugs
- Latex
- Mold
- Sinus infection
- Seasonal

Typical symptoms include:

- Runny or stuffy nose, sneezing
- Wheezing, shortness of breath
- Cough
- Rashes
- Fatigue
- Headache
- Nausea, vomiting
- Fever
- Headache
- Anaphylaxis (rare but severe)

For proper treatment, the first step is to get evaluated by a board-certified allergist-immunologist. A skin or blood test may be performed to determine your precise type of allergy. Treatment typically involves medication or immunotherapy.

Asthma

Asthma is a condition that causes your airways to narrow, swell, and create extra mucus. Symptoms include coughing, wheezing, shortness of breath, and chest tightness. For asthmatic athletes, these symptoms can pose some challenges. Asthma inhalers are commonly used to relax the muscles that tighten around the airways. Short-acting bronchodilator inhalers used prior to and during exercise can relieve symptoms. Exercise-induced asthma is often worse when the air is cold and dry. Unfortunately, many of the asthma inhalers marketed in the United States contain short- and long-acting beta-2 agonists, which are included on WADA's list of prohibited substances. If you require the use of an inhaler, it's important that you know your sport's anti-doping rules in order to determine if you'll need a therapeutic use exemption (TUE). Athletes can visit GlobalDRO.com to learn about the prohibited status of specific medications.

Diabetes

Diabetes mellitus refers to a group of diseases that affects how your body uses blood sugar or glucose. In chapter 3, we learned that glucose is a vital source of energy for your muscles, liver, and brain. Type 1 and type 2 diabetes are lifelong conditions, whereas prediabetes and gestational diabetes are reversible. In type 1 diabetes, the immune system attacks and destroys your own insulin-producing cells in the pancreas, leaving your body with little to no insulin. This causes glucose to build up in the bloodstream instead of going to cells. A common barrier to exercise for people with type 1 diabetes is the fear of hypoglycemia or the difficulty of knowing how exercise will affect blood glucose. In type 2 diabetes, cells become resistant to the action of insulin. Less glucose enters the cells, and sugar builds up to harmful levels in the bloodstream. Type 2 diabetes is strongly linked to being overweight. If you have diabetes, take time to learn how the energy demands of your sport or exercise regimen will affect blood glucose. Understanding how your diabetes influences your active lifestyle will make it safe for you to participate in sports. The disease usually demands that you continuously monitor blood glucose while adjusting diet and insulin as needed. (Diabetic athletes should also always carry a form of diabetes identification.) Take comfort in knowing that you'll still get to participate in the events you enjoy.

Autoimmune Diseases

The immune system normally guards against bacteria and viruses when it senses foreign invaders. But with an autoimmune disease, your immune system mistakenly attacks the healthy cells in your body. There are more than 80 different autoimmune diseases.

Common autoimmune diseases:

- Type 1 diabetes
- Rheumatoid arthritis (RA)
- Psoriasis
- Multiple sclerosis
- Lupus
- Crohn's disease
- Addison's disease
- Fibromyalgia
- Graves' disease
- Ulcerative colitis
- Sjögren's syndrome
- Hashimoto's thyroiditis
- Myasthenia gravis
- Vasculitis
- Celiac disease

Although each disease has its own symptoms, typical complaints include fatigue, achy muscles, skin rashes, swelling, and a low-grade fever. Exercise is a bit of a two-edged sword: Sometimes it can reduce inflammation, but other times it can exacerbate pain. Listen to your body and communicate with your coaches. Recognize the activities that help control symptoms, and modify your training during flare-ups. If you feel too exhausted to exercise, let your body recover with a casual walk, and don't feel guilty about missing a structured workout.

Cancer

You probably know someone who has been affected by cancer. Cancer is a disease caused by changes in the genes that control the functioning of cells. There are more than 100 types of cancer. Normally, healthy cells grow and divide to form new cells as the body needs them. When these types of cells grow old or become damaged, they die and new cells take their place. With cancer, old or damaged cells don't die. Instead the cells keep growing and dividing. As a result, the cells keep doubling, forming a tumor that can continue to grow in size. When a cancer is malignant, it can spread to nearby tissue via the bloodstream or lymph system. Side effects of cancer treatment (i.e., chemotherapy, radiation) include lack of appetite, diarrhea, constipation, fatigue, pain, and insomnia. Unfortunately, these side effects often affect the ability to consistently follow a training plan. If you have cancer and want to exercise, take into account the type and stage of your disease. Be sure to factor in time for treatment, as well as your energy and strength levels.

Exercise plays a favorable role in cancer prevention treatment and survivorship. Benefits include:

- Improved quality of life
- Improved physical functioning
- Increased blood flow, which lowers the risk of blood clots
- Better self-esteem
- Higher energy levels
- Increased social contacts
- Improved body composition
- Improved muscle strength and endurance
- Improved immune function
- Improved cardiovascular fitness
- Decreased risk of anxiety or depression
- Reduced nausea
- Decrease in muscle atrophy

13

CHAPTER

Body and Brain

If you experience pre-competition nerves, you're not alone. Athletes often talk about an elevated heart rate, butterflies in their stomach, tight muscles, phantom pains and sickness, anxiety, and a lack of appetite. These pre-event jitters are proof that physical training isn't the only factor for a successful competition. Just as you've trained your muscles, you must also train your mind so your body can perform to its full ability. Mental training, such as meditation, positive affirmations, breathing, and visualization techniques, is just as important as physical training. These practices can help develop a brain-body connection so you can maintain a high level of motivation, increase your confidence, and improve your concentration. By learning to remove distractions, you can better manage competition anxiety, nerves, and emotions. The relationship between thoughts and actions is complex. Building brain power—often with the help of a sports psychologist—may be the key to unlocking your athletic potential.

Negative Self-Talk

Most athletes don't realize that the voice inside their heads can often be nasty and negative. Have you ever found yourself thinking "I know I'm not going to do well today" before an upcoming competition? This negative self-talk raises your stress levels by decreasing your self-confidence. So what can you do with all this self-directed negativity? First, understand that self-talk is normal. While a little self-criticism can be a good thing, there's a big difference between "I need to work on my shooting skills" and "I suck at basketball." Much of your thinking may be inaccurate or exaggerated, so the key is to learn how to react to your thoughts in a calm and positive way. The next time you hear a negative thought in your head, ask yourself if you have any evidence to back it up. Next, consider another way to look at the situation. Rather than believing what you hear in your head, conquer it with positive affirmations. The great thing about self-talk is that it can't predict the future. Even if you *think* you are not having a good race, you may still be able to put together a great performance. If your negative self-talk is so severe that you can't get self-defeating thoughts out of your head, a sports psychologist can help. He or she can provide a safe place to sort out why these thoughts developed and how to create constructive thoughts to foster athletic success. Negative self-talk can increase anxiety under pressure—here are some tips to help reduce the pre-competition nerves:

1. Be aware, but not afraid, of situations that stress you out and make you feel most anxious, nervous, or scared.

2. Focus on the process or task at hand and not on the outcome. Put your energy into the factors you can control and stay in the moment.

3. Go into your event with a no-expectations/no-pressure mind-set. Get excited about the unknown.

4. Avoid people who suck the energy out of you. Surround yourself with energy givers.

5. Create positive mantras and affirmations to help you get through uncomfortable and difficult situations.

6. Practice good breathing skills.

7. Visualize success.

Concentration

Loss of concentration is often blamed for poor performance in sports. Concentration requires the ability to exert deliberate mental energy and positive self-talk to a given situation while focusing on the "doing" instead of the "how to do." Concentrating requires that you focus only on the present moment. Take, for example, a biathlon, which involves cross-country skiing and rifle shooting. During the shooting component, the biathlete must maintain intense focus on their target skills and not on the next lap of cross-country skiing. Different types of concentration are needed for different sports. Tennis demands quick, in-the-moment concentration, while long-duration sports, such as the Ironman, require sustained focus and concentration. Cheers from fans, background noise, weather conditions, and even being in the presence of other athletes can distract you and cause concentration to wane. To improve concentration, athletes must train the brain to switch on and off. Doing visualization exercises, establishing a routine or ritual, and mentally removing distractions can help discourage distraction. Put energy into what's in your control. Your mind is a muscle that needs to be trained. Try this exercise to improve your mental focus—it's a lot harder than you think!

Clock Concentration

1. Sit directly in front of a clock with a second hand.

2. Follow the second hand with your eyes as it goes around and around.

3. Keep this up for as long as you can (start with one minute and work up to 5 minutes). Think of nothing else but watching the second hand.

4. Don't look away, and avoid being distracted by random thoughts, sensations in the body, or other sounds in the room.

If you fail at first, don't get discouraged. It's natural for the mind to wander, but with practice, you can improve your concentration and self-control.

Visualization and Mindfulness

There's great power in being mindful, in visualizing success and learning to be "in the zone" or "in a state of flow." When visualization is used correctly, athletes can start an event believing they have already succeeded. How is this possible? It's because they have visualized victory long before the actual competition. The mindful athlete can clear out the clutter and accept things as they are without judgment. Downhill skiers, ice skaters, and gymnasts often use these practices, developing and mastering the skills over time. Although visualization can seem quite simple, it's natural to think of all the obstacles that could be in your way. But instead of creating mental barriers and difficulties, see yourself victorious. Visualize your next winning goal or an impeccable performance. While it's important to stay positive during visualization, you should also envision unfavorable situations that require problem-solving skills and a calm demeanor. Ultimately, if you can't picture yourself achieving a goal, there's a good chance you won't achieve it. Get into the habit of creating a positive vision of success every day. While many athletes employ sports psychologists to help them with their visualizations, you can also do it on your own. Try this simple visualization technique for 5 to 15 minutes each day in the weeks before a competition:

1. Sit or lie down in a quiet room with no distractions.

2. Close your eyes and imagine, in vivid detail, your upcoming event or competition. Visualize yourself scoring a goal, setting a personal-best time, or accomplishing a move you've never mastered before. What is the weather, scenery, and atmosphere like?

3. Be sure to use all of your senses. Imagine the course, how your body feels, and even the sounds and smells around you.

4. Mentally rehearse specific skills under pressure, especially the uncomfortable situations. Without getting caught up in unconstructive thoughts and emotions, go through all of the rituals or routines you will use to create event-day success.

PART FOUR

Recipes for Success

As you learned earlier in this book, it's important to think about what you eat before, during, and after exercise, as well as on rest days. But let's get real—the last thing any of us wants to do after a grueling workout is toil away in the kitchen. Meal planning can ease some of the burden while helping you feel confident about meeting your daily nutritional needs. It can also ensure that you're getting enough of the right nutrients, at the right times. In the next few chapters you'll find delicious, nutritionally balanced recipes. Most are easy-to-follow recipes that come together quickly, with easy-to-find ingredients. They're intended to deliver the nutrients you need to help you perform at your best. The chapters are organized into recipes for before, during, and after exercise or competition, and for rest days to help you apply the concept of nutrient timing, but I encourage you to work these performance-focused recipes into your daily routine, whenever you feel they work best in your lifestyle.

14

CHAPTER

Recipes for Before Exercise or Competition

APRICOT-COCONUT GRANOLA 136

BAKED BLUEBERRY OATMEAL 137

BLUEBERRY-STUFFED CHALLAH FRENCH TOAST 138

CARROT CAKE MUFFINS 139

CINNAMON QUINOA BOWL 140

OVER-EASY GRITS BOWL 141

SWEET POTATO PROTEIN PANCAKES 142

APRICOT-COCONUT GRANOLA

VEGETARIAN Granola is the perfect energy-dense food to give your muscles quality fuel before exercise. Since many store-bought versions have high amounts of added sugar and oils, it's better to make your own. It's easy, delicious, and inexpensive—and you can control the amount of sugar and fat. Granola can be a meal or a snack, as well as a topping for yogurt, oatmeal, or a smoothie bowl.

Yield: 7 cups
Prep: 10 minutes
Cook: 35 minutes

3 cups oats
1½ cups shredded coconut
1½ cups sliced almonds
¾ teaspoon salt
2 tablespoons butter, melted (or 3 tablespoons coconut oil, melted, to make it vegan)
¾ cup honey (or ¾ cup maple syrup and 2 tablespoons sugar, to make it vegan)
½ cup dried apricots, chopped
½ cup dried cherries or cranberries), chopped

1. Preheat the oven to 325°.

2. In a large bowl, combine the oats, coconut, almonds, and salt and toss.

3. In a small bowl, combine the melted butter and honey and mix.

4. Add the honey mixture to the oats mixture and toss until evenly combined.

5. Spread the mixture evenly on a parchment paper–lined baking sheet.

6. Bake for 25 minutes, or until the granola is light golden brown. Stir with a spatula every 10 minutes to keep the edges from burning.

7. Remove from the oven and add the apricots and dried cherries. Toss again.

8. Turn off the oven and put the granola back in the oven for 10 minutes.

9. Let cool and serve.

Storage: Keeps for 2 weeks in an airtight container.

Per Serving (1/2 cup): Calories: 279; Saturated Fat: 7g; Total Fat: 13g; Protein: 5g; Total Carbs: 39g; Fiber: 5g; Sodium: 130mg

BAKED BLUEBERRY OATMEAL

DAIRY-FREE, VEGAN High in complex carbohydrates, with a low glycemic index, oatmeal provides a sustained release of energy to give you a long-lasting boost. Blueberries are nutrient-packed powerhouses. This baked oatmeal is rich in antioxidants and vitamin C, making it an excellent pre-workout meal. It's also great as a snack to help boost the immune system. I like it served warm and topped with yogurt and a drizzle of syrup, but it's also good at room temperature.

Yield: 15 servings
Prep: 20 minutes
Cook: 45 minutes

2 tablespoons flaxseed meal

¼ cup plus 2 tablespoons water

⅔ cup chopped pecans

2 cups old-fashioned oats (use gluten-free oats to make it gluten-free)

2 teaspoons ground cinnamon

1 teaspoon baking powder

½ teaspoon salt

1¾ cups almond milk

⅓ cup maple syrup

3 tablespoons coconut oil, melted

2 teaspoons vanilla extract

2½ cups fresh (or frozen) blueberries, divided

1. Make flax eggs by mixing together the flaxseed meal with the water. Let it sit in the refrigerator for 15 minutes, or until thick.

2. Preheat the oven to 375°F. Grease a 9-inch-square baking dish.

3. In a medium bowl, combine the pecans, oats, cinnamon, baking powder, and salt.

4. In another medium bowl, combine the almond milk, maple syrup, flax egg, coconut oil, and vanilla. Whisk until combined. It's okay if the coconut oil solidifies when you add it to the wet ingredients; simply break up any larger pieces with your hands.

5. Spread 2 cups of blueberries in the prepared baking dish. Cover the fruit with the oats mixture, then pour the wet ingredients on top.

6. Lightly shake the baking dish to fully soak the oats, then gently pat down.

7. Spread the remaining ½ cup of berries on top.

8. Bake for 45 minutes, or until the top is golden.

9. Remove the baked oatmeal from the oven and let cool for a few minutes before serving.

Storage: Keeps for 5 days covered in the refrigerator. Eat the baked oatmeal cold or pre-portion into single servings and heat in the microwave.

Ingredient tip: For more protein and fat, use cow's milk in place of the almond milk and 2 large eggs in place of the flax eggs.

Per Serving: Calories: 147; Saturated Fat: 3g; Total Fat: 8g; Protein: 2g; Total Carbs: 19g; Fiber: 3g; Sodium: 130mg

BLUEBERRY-STUFFED CHALLAH FRENCH TOAST

VEGETARIAN French toast is a breakfast menu favorite, and for good reason. It's hard to resist a thick, fluffy, egg-coated piece of bread topped with a drizzle of warm maple syrup and a sprinkle of powdered sugar. French toast is the ultimate comfort breakfast meal, and it's also a great performance meal for athletes—thanks to the combination of carbohydrates and protein. This recipe is very quick to make—ideal before a long training session or endurance competition.

Yield: 2 servings
Prep: 10 minutes
Cook: 10 minutes

1 egg

¼ cup low-fat milk

¼ teaspoon sugar

2 to 3 tablespoons whipped cream cheese (adjust amount to your liking)

4 slices challah bread

½ cup fresh blueberries, plus more for garnish

2 teaspoons butter

Warm maple syrup, for topping

1. In a shallow bowl, whisk together the egg, milk, and sugar.

2. Spread the cream cheese on all four bread slices. Top two of the slices with the blueberries and close the sandwiches. Gently press around the crust to seal.

3. Heat a large skillet over medium to medium-high heat and melt the butter to coat the pan.

4. Dip each sandwich in egg mixture on both sides, and cook until golden brown, also on both sides.

5. Top with warm maple syrup and more blueberries and serve immediately.

Ingredient tip: Make sure the bread is cut at least 1 inch thick. (If the bread is too thin, it won't hold together when dipped in the batter.) Brioche, French bread, and Pullman loaf are spongy and sturdy enough to maintain their shape during soaking. If blueberries aren't in season, try frozen blueberries that have been thawed in the refrigerator overnight (microwaving can make frozen berries soggy), or substitute with strawberries or blackberries.

Per Serving: Calories: 429; Saturated Fat: 6g; Total Fat: 15g; Protein: 13g; Total Carbs: 66g; Fiber: 3g; Sodium: 422mg

CARROT CAKE MUFFINS

DAIRY-FREE, VEGETARIAN I love carrot cake, maybe because it's a cake made with a vegetable. This classic dessert is so incredibly moist, tender, and full of flavor that it's hard to resist. Because the typical carrot cake recipe calls for cream cheese frosting and lots of sugar and butter, it can be extremely high in calories and fat. But don't fret: My recipe uses applesauce in place of most of the oil. I guarantee you'll feel great about these healthy on-the-go-muffins.

Yield: 12 muffins
Prep: 20 minutes
Cook: 20 minutes

¼ cup unsweetened applesauce

1½ teaspoons canola oil

½ cup brown sugar

1 egg

1 teaspoon vanilla extract

¾ cup finely chopped carrots (3 to 4 medium carrots)

¼ teaspoon salt

1 teaspoon ground cinnamon

¼ teaspoon nutmeg

1½ teaspoons baking powder

1 cup all-purpose flour

¼ cup walnuts, chopped

1. Preheat the oven to 350°F. Line a muffin pan with 12 muffin liners.

2. In a large bowl, using a handheld mixer or in a stand mixer, beat together the applesauce, oil, and brown sugar on low speed until combined. Mix in the egg and vanilla. Add the carrots and mix until combined.

3. Add the salt, cinnamon, nutmeg, baking powder, and flour to the applesauce mixture and continue beating on low speed (or stir with a wooden spoon).

4. Divide the batter evenly between cups in the prepared muffin pan (a #40 cookie scoop works well for portioning).

5. Top the batter in each muffin cup with a few chopped walnuts.

6. Bake for 17 to 20 minutes, or just until a toothpick inserted in the center comes out mostly clean.

7. Let the muffins cool on a wire rack.

Storage: Store the muffins in an airtight container for 1 week, or freeze in a heavy-duty freezer bag for up to 2 months.

Recipe tip: To keep the muffins from sticking to the inside of the liners, let them cool completely before removing from the wrappers. Alternatively, use nonstick liners.

Per Serving (1 muffin): Calories: 105; Saturated Fat: 0g; Total Fat: 3g; Protein: 2g; Total Carbs: 18g; Fiber: 1g; Sodium: 127mg

CINNAMON QUINOA BOWL

GLUTEN-FREE, VEGETARIAN Quinoa (pronounced KEEN-wah) is often called an "ancient grain," but—surprise—it's a seed. Rich in iron, manganese, magnesium, B vitamins, and fiber, quinoa is also a complete protein, which means it contains all nine essential amino acids. And cinnamon may help reduce inflammation and ease muscle soreness. I suggest you make an extra serving or two of this bowl for a post-workout snack.

Yield: 2 servings
Prep: 5 minutes
Cook: 20 minutes

1 cup quinoa

2 tablespoons chopped
  raw pecans

1½ teaspoons butter

½ teaspoon ground cinnamon,
  plus more for topping

Pinch salt

1½ tablespoons maple syrup

1 tablespoon dried
  cranberries, chopped

¼ teaspoon chia
  seeds (optional)

1. In a medium saucepan, bring 2 cups of water to a boil. Stir in the quinoa, then immediately reduce the heat to low. Cover and simmer for about 15 minutes, or until the liquid is completely absorbed. Use a fork to fluff the quinoa.

2. Put the pecans in a separate medium saucepan over medium heat and stir until fragrant and browned, about 5 minutes.

3. Add the butter, cinnamon, and salt and stir until well combined.

4. Stir in 1 cup of the cooked quinoa. (One cup dry quinoa yields about 3 cups cooked. Reserve the leftover quinoa for another meal; see tip below.)

5. Remove the pan from the heat and stir in the maple syrup.

6. Transfer the mixture to a bowl and top with the dried cranberries and chia seeds (if using).

7. Serve immediately.

Make-ahead tip: Prepare a big batch of quinoa in advance and store in the refrigerator in an airtight container to use for other meals during the week. Cooked quinoa will keep for 1 week in the refrigerator.

Per Serving: Calories: 253; Saturated Fat: 3g; Total Fat: 10g; Protein: 5g; Total Carbs: 38g; Fiber: 4g; Sodium: 154mg

OVER-EASY GRITS BOWL

GLUTEN-FREE, VEGETARIAN Grits are made of hominy, which are small, dried kernels of corn. Oatmeal gets praised for being the perfect pre-workout food because of its high carb content, but just one cup of grits is actually even higher in carbs. Remember, carbohydrates can help keep your muscles energized throughout strenuous activities. Athletes with sensitive stomachs may find it easier to digest grits because of the low fiber content. If you only have an hour or less to digest this meal, I suggest omitting the egg and topping with only a sprinkle of cheese to lower the fat content.

Yield: 1 serving
Prep: 5 minutes
Cook: 5 minutes

¼ cup instant grits
1 cup water
Pinch salt
½ teaspoon butter
1 egg
¼ cup shredded sharp
  Cheddar cheese
⅛ teaspoon garlic powder
Freshly ground black pepper
¼ teaspoon dried parsley

1. Put the instant grits, water, and salt in a microwave-safe bowl and stir to combine. Microwave for 2½ to 3 minutes.

2. Meanwhile, in a nonstick skillet over medium heat, melt the butter until foamy. Gently break the egg into the pan and cook until the white is firm and the yolk begins to thicken but isn't hard.

3. Gently slide a spatula under the egg and flip. Cook until the egg reaches your desired doneness.

4. Remove the grits from the microwave and stir in the cheese, garlic powder, and pepper, stirring until the cheese is melted.

5. Slide the cooked egg on top of the grits mixture and top with the dried parsley.

6. Chop the egg into the grits mixture.

Ingredient tip: Add cooked lean turkey sausage to the bowl if you want to increase protein and fat content.

Per Serving: Calories: 267; Saturated Fat: 8g; Total Fat: 16g; Protein: 15g; Total Carbs: 18g; Fiber: 1g; Sodium: 788mg

SWEET POTATO PROTEIN PANCAKES

GLUTEN-FREE, VEGETARIAN These satisfying, protein-packed pancakes are a great way to start your day when you have a workout scheduled. You can also enjoy them as an on-the-go breakfast meal or snack. Rich in protein, calcium, and sodium, cottage cheese is a great all-around health food to help build muscle, boost immunity, and strengthen bones. Make sure to choose a cottage cheese brand that contains fat (ex. 2%) and limited ingredients. These pancakes are so tasty, you won't even realize you're eating cottage cheese.

Yield: 10 (4½-inch) pancakes
Prep: 15 minutes
Cook: 15 minutes

2 sweet potatoes
1 cup gluten-free rolled oats
1 cup 2% cottage cheese
2 large eggs
4 large egg whites
1 teaspoon baking powder
1 teaspoon vanilla extract
¼ teaspoon ground cinnamon
¼ teaspoon ground nutmeg
Nonstick cooking spray
Maple syrup, for serving
  (optional)

1. Pierce the potatoes five or six times with a fork and microwave for 5 to 8 minutes, rotating halfway through.

2. Place the oats in a food processor and grind until they make a fine oat flour. Transfer to a large bowl and set aside.

3. Place the cottage cheese in the food processor and process until smooth. Add to the bowl with the oats and stir well.

4. Scoop the sweet potato flesh into the food processor and process until smooth. Add to the bowl with the oats and cottage cheese and stir well.

5. Add the eggs, egg whites, baking powder, vanilla, cinnamon, and nutmeg to the cottage cheese mixture and stir well. If you prefer a thinner pancake, add a little water to achieve your desired consistency.

6. Heat a skillet or griddle over medium heat and spray with nonstick cooking spray.

7. Using a ½-cup measuring cup, portion the batter onto the skillet or griddle. Cook the pancakes until bubbles form and begin to burst in the center, about 4 minutes. Flip with a spatula and cook until done, 3 to 4 minutes.

8. Serve with maple syrup (if desired).

Storage: Wrap leftover pancakes in plastic wrap and refrigerate for up to 4 days, or freeze in a storage bag for up to a month. When you are ready to eat, pop the pancakes in the toaster until heated through.

Make-ahead tip: To save some time, cook the sweet potatoes in advance. You can freeze the cooked potatoes in a resealable bag and thaw in the refrigerator or microwave before using.

Per Serving (2 pancakes): Calories: 192; Saturated Fat: 1g; Total Fat: 4g; Protein: 13g; Total Carbs: 25g; Fiber: 3g; Sodium: 333mg

15

Recipes for During and After Exercise

PEANUT BUTTER PROTEIN BALLS 144

ALMOND BUTTER AND APPLE SANDWICHES 145

PEANUT BUTTER PRETZEL BALLS 146

PERFECT PUMPKIN ENERGY BALLS 147

BERRY-CHERRY SMOOTHIE 148

ORGANIC CHICKPEA FUSILLI WITH
GOAT CHEESE 149

CRUST-FREE SPINACH, MUSHROOM,
AND CHEESE QUICHE 150

SLOW COOKER SWEET POTATO QUINOA CURRY 151

BUENO BREAKFAST BURRITO 152

PEANUT BUTTER PROTEIN BALLS

GLUTEN-FREE, VEGETARIAN These no-bake peanut butter bites make for a perfect energy-boosting treat when you're exercising, traveling, at the office, or in school. Super easy to assemble, they offer a satiating combination of protein, carbs, and fat—just right when you need to recharge during an all-day event. For young athletes, these protein balls are a great fuel source to help maintain energy levels during training and games. Plus, they're a much healthier alternative to heavily sweetened, processed snacks.

Yield: 30 balls
Prep: 20 minutes

1 cup old-fashioned rolled oats

¼ cup chia seeds

10 pitted dates

½ cup creamy peanut butter

1 scoop vanilla whey protein powder (18 to 25g protein)

¼ cup water

2 teaspoons vanilla extract

1 teaspoon ground cinnamon

1. In a food processor, pulse the oats and chia seeds until they reach an almost flour-like consistency.

2. Add the dates, peanut butter, protein powder, vanilla extract, and cinnamon to the food processor. Pulse until well blended.

3. Slowly add the water to the food processor and blend until the mixture begins to stick together. You may need to add more or less water depending on the dough consistency.

4. Transfer the mixture to a large bowl. Form into 1-inch balls and place on a parchment paper–lined baking sheet. Let set for 5 minutes before eating or preparing for storage (see tip below).

Storage: Refrigerate the protein balls in an airtight container for a week, or freeze in a freezer bag for up to a month. If frozen, let thaw at room temperature for 15 to 30 minutes or warm in the microwave for 15 to 30 seconds before eating.

Per Serving (1 ball): Calories: 54; Saturated Fat: 1g; Total Fat: 3g; Protein: 2g; Total Carbs: 5g; Fiber: 1g; Sodium: 24mg

ALMOND BUTTER AND APPLE SANDWICHES

DAIRY-FREE, GLUTEN-FREE, PALEO, VEGETARIAN These delightful sandwiches are sure to please anyone who loves apples and nut butter. The combination of ingredients will help prevent a rumbling stomach during all-day tournaments. The addition of honey, flaxseed, and coconut makes the typical apple and nut butter combo much more delicious. The lemon juice is used to prevent the apple from browning if you don't plan to eat right away. If you're taking these sandwiches on the go, chill them first and then wrap in aluminum foil. You can omit the shredded coconut to avoid a mess when eating on the go.

Yield: 8 sandwiches
Prep: 10 minutes

2 large apples, cored
Juice of ½ lemon
¼ cup almond butter
1 tablespoon honey
2 teaspoons milled
    flaxseed (optional)
3 tablespoons shredded
    unsweetened coconut
Ground cinnamon,
    for sprinkling

1. Slice the apples horizontally into 16 disks. The apple disks will form the base of the sandwiches, so keep similarly sized disks paired together.

2. Put the lemon juice in a small bowl and dip both sides of the apple slices in the juice to help prevent browning.

3. Spread half of the apple slices with a thin layer of almond butter. Drizzle the honey over the almond butter. Sprinkle milled flaxseed (if using) over the honey.

4. Place the remaining apple slices on top to make sandwiches. Gently press together.

5. Put the shredded coconut on a small plate. Roll the sandwiches in the coconut so that it sticks to the almond butter.

6. Sprinkle with cinnamon and enjoy immediately, or refrigerate to set.

Storage: Store in an airtight container in the refrigerator (or in a cooler on game days) for up to 3 days.

Per Serving (2 sandwiches): Calories: 200; Saturated Fat: 3g; Total Fat: 12g; Protein: 4g; Total Carbs: 23g; Fiber: 5g; Sodium: 1mg

PEANUT BUTTER PRETZEL BALLS

DAIRY-FREE, VEGETARIAN Ask any endurance athlete and she'll tell you that flavor fatigue is a recurring problem during training. Relying on sugary sports drinks to meet hourly nutrition needs while training and racing gets tiresome. These savory pretzel balls are the perfect counterbalance to that sweetness. Low in fiber and fat, yet high in sodium and carbs, pretzels are the ideal training food. And when you pair them with peanut butter, you have the perfect combination of salty and savory. For athletes participating in long-duration practices or competitions, these peanut butter pretzel balls provide a great source of sustainable energy. Plus, they are a real-food alternative to heavily processed sports bars that you can enjoy any time of day.

Yield: 24 balls
Prep: 15 minutes

2 cups bite-size pretzels
¾ cup creamy peanut butter
2½ tablespoons honey
½ teaspoon ground cinnamon

1. Put the pretzels in a resealable plastic bag. Crush with a rolling pin or pound with a meat tenderizer/mallet until finely crushed but not too powdery.

2. In a medium bowl, stir together the peanut butter, honey, and cinnamon. Stir in the crushed pretzels until well combined.

3. Use a tablespoon to scoop the mixture and roll into 24 balls. Transfer to a parchment paper–lined baking sheet.

4. Freeze on the baking sheet for 10 minutes to set.

Storage: Store in an airtight container in the refrigerator for up to a week. Or store in the freezer, in a heavy-duty freezer bag, for up to 1 month.

Ingredient tip: Mix in ¼ cup of your favorite chopped, dried fruit to change things up. You can also add chocolate chips (but they may melt and make a mess in the heat).

Per Serving (1 ball): Calories: 67; Saturated Fat: 1g; Total Fat: 4g; Protein: 2g; Total Carbs: 6g; Fiber: 1g; Sodium: 63mg

PERFECT PUMPKIN ENERGY BALLS

DAIRY-FREE, VEGAN Pumpkin is one power-packed food. This fruit—no, it's not a vegetable—packs 400 milligrams of potassium in a 1-cup serving. These energy balls are a good source of carbohydrates with a little fat. They're super delicious and easy to digest when exercising at low intensity, especially in the cold winter months. They're also convenient to pack for long bike rides and hikes, as well as trips to the gym.

Yield: 12 balls
Prep: 12 minutes, plus
30 minutes to chill

1 cup pitted Medjool dates
  (10 to 12 large dates)
1 cup old-fashioned oats
¼ cup walnuts
¼ cup pumpkin purée
1 tablespoon maple syrup
1 tablespoon chia seeds
  (or ground flaxseed)
2 teaspoons pumpkin pie spice
½ teaspoon salt

1. In a food processor, process the dates, oats, walnuts, pumpkin purée, maple syrup, chia seeds, pumpkin pie spice, and salt until thoroughly mixed. Transfer the mixture to a bowl.

2. Using a cookie scoop or spoon, scoop the mixture into balls and place on a parchment paper–lined baking sheet.

3. Refrigerate on the baking sheet for at least 30 minutes before serving.

Storage: Store in an airtight container in the refrigerator for up to 2 weeks, or freeze in an airtight container or freezer bag for up to 2 months.

Ingredient tip: Make your own pumpkin pie spice: Combine 3 tablespoons ground cinnamon, 2 teaspoons ground ginger, 2 teaspoons nutmeg, 1½ teaspoons ground allspice, and 1½ teaspoons ground cloves. Also, because these energy balls are so easy to make, I suggest doubling the recipe to make a batch for your favorite training partner.

Per Serving (1 ball): Calories: 120; Saturated Fat: 0g; Total Fat: 2g; Protein: 2g; Total Carbs: 24g; Fiber: 3g; Sodium: 102mg

BERRY-CHERRY SMOOTHIE

VEGETARIAN Nutritional science research suggests that antioxidant-rich cherries have powerful anti-inflammatory benefits that help with muscle recovery and pain relief. This refreshingly delicious smoothie recipe combines flavors of both tart and sweet cherries. If you don't have an appetite for solid food post-workout, this is your go-to drink.

Yield: 2 servings
Prep: 5 minutes

1 cup sweet cherries, pitted and stems removed

½ cup 100% tart cherry juice

1 cup fresh strawberries, hulled

¼ cup freshly squeezed orange juice

½ cup vanilla yogurt

2 tablespoons honey

2 cups ice cubes

Nutmeg, for garnish (optional)

1. In a blender, combine all of the ingredients except the nutmeg and blend until smooth.

2. Pour into glasses and sprinkle with nutmeg, if using.

Ingredient tip: If sweet cherries aren't in season, you can use thawed frozen cherries. If you don't have a cherry pitter, use an unbent paper clip or a toothpick to remove the pits. To make this smoothie vegan, use dairy-free yogurt and substitute maple syrup for the honey.

Per Serving: Calories: 254; Saturated Fat: 1g; Total Fat: 1g; Protein: 7g; Total Carbs: 59g; Fiber: 4g; Sodium: 58mg

ORGANIC CHICKPEA FUSILLI WITH GOAT CHEESE

GLUTEN-FREE, VEGETARIAN Pasta has reigned as a go-to pre-competition meal for good reason. It's quick and easy to make and a great source of carbs. Plus, traditional pasta is easy to digest before a competition. For a healthier alternative to semolina flour, try plant-based pasta varieties, such as bean, pea, lentil, edamame, or chickpea. They're packed with fiber and protein, and can be enjoyed anytime, even outside of competitions or events. Look for these pasta options online or in the gluten-free section of your grocery store.

Yield: 4 servings
Prep: 15 minutes
Cook: 20 minutes

8 ounces organic
   chickpea fusilli
2 tablespoons olive oil
2 cups chopped baby
   tomatoes
1 cup chopped white onion
8 ounces sliced mushrooms
1 large garlic clove,
   finely chopped
½ cup dry roasted pepitas
½ cup chopped fresh basil
Pinch of salt
2 cups baby spinach
1 tablespoon freshly
   squeezed lemon juice
½ cup goat cheese, crumbled

1. Cook the fusilli according to the package directions.

2. While the pasta is cooking, heat the olive oil in a large skillet over medium heat.

3. Add the chopped tomatoes, onion, and mushrooms. Gently toss and sauté until lightly browned and softened, 8 to 10 minutes.

4. Add the garlic, pepitas, basil, salt, spinach, and lemon juice. Gently toss and cook for 2 minutes. Remove from the heat.

5. Add the cooked pasta to the veggie mix.

6. Top with the goat cheese.

Recipe tip: To keep yourself organized while making this dish, try using a muffin tin to hold tiny ingredients like herbs and spices and small bowls for the other ingredients. Cut up extra veggies while you're at it to use for salads and stir-fry dishes later in the week.

Per Serving: Calories: 435; Saturated Fat: 4g; Total Fat: 19g; Protein: 21g; Total Carbs: 51g; Fiber: 9g; Sodium: 166mg

CRUST-FREE SPINACH, MUSHROOM, AND CHEESE QUICHE

GLUTEN-FREE, VEGETARIAN Fast and easy meals are important, but having leftovers can be a game-changer, especially when you're crunched for time. Quiche is a convenient, high-protein option because you don't have to be a skilled chef to make it and there's always extra for a future meal. Plus, you can customize it however you like. I left out the crust to highlight the eggs and veggies, but you can add more carbs by adding a store-bought crust, or serve with toast, rice, or potatoes.

Yield: 6 servings
Prep: 20 minutes
Cook: 45 minutes

1 (10-ounce) box chopped frozen spinach, thawed
1 teaspoon olive oil
2 garlic cloves, minced
8 ounces sliced mushrooms, halved
Salt, to taste
Freshly ground black pepper, to taste
Nonstick cooking spray
⅓ cup feta cheese, crumbled
4 large eggs
1 cup milk
½ teaspoon garlic salt
¼ cup grated Parmesan cheese
½ cup shredded mozzarella cheese

1. Preheat the oven to 350°F.

2. Squeeze the excess water from the spinach.

3. In a medium skillet, heat the olive oil over medium-high heat.

4. Add the garlic and cook for about 1 minute, or until fragrant. Add the mushrooms, season with salt and pepper, and sauté until the mushrooms are tender. Drain the excess liquid from the cooked mushrooms.

5. Coat a 9-inch glass pie dish with cooking spray. Place the spinach in the bottom of the pie dish. Top with the sautéed mushrooms, followed by the crumbled feta cheese.

6. In a medium bowl, whisk together the eggs, milk, garlic salt, and Parmesan cheese. Pour the egg mixture over the vegetables and feta in the pie dish. Top with the mozzarella cheese.

7. Place the pie dish on a baking sheet and bake in the oven for 45 to 50 minutes, or until the quiche has set and the top is golden brown.

8. Cut into six slices and serve.

Recipe tip: Let the quiche cool completely on the counter before covering with foil or placing in an airtight container and refrigerating. Traditionally, quiche is served at room temperature, but if it's left outside for more than two hours, the ingredients can create an ideal environment for bacteria to thrive.

Per Serving: Calories: 159; Saturated Fat: 5g; Total Fat: 10g; Protein: 12g; Total Carbs: 10g; Fiber: 2g; Sodium: 550mg

SLOW COOKER SWEET POTATO QUINOA CURRY

DAIRY-FREE, GLUTEN-FREE, VEGAN Slow cookers are undoubtedly convenient because they save you a lot of time. Before you leave for work or school, you can put all your ingredients in the pot, and when you come home, you'll have a meal already prepared for you, plus leftovers! Packed with herbs, spices, and vegetables, this meal is flavorful, satiating, and nutritious, and it's sure to boost your immune system after a tough workout or competition.

Yield: 6 servings
Prep: 45 minutes
Cook: 3 to 4 hours

1 (28-ounce) can plain diced tomatoes, undrained

1 large or 2 small sweet potatoes, peeled and chopped (about 3 cups)

2 cups broccoli crowns, cut into bite-size pieces

1 (15-ounce) can chickpeas, drained and rinsed

2 (14.5-ounce) cans light coconut milk

1 cup water

1 small onion, chopped

½ cup quinoa, rinsed

3 garlic cloves, minced

1 tablespoon reduced-sodium soy sauce (or gluten-free tamari)

1 tablespoon grated peeled fresh ginger

1 teaspoon ground turmeric

½ teaspoon ground cumin

¼ teaspoon red pepper flakes

Chopped fresh cilantro, for garnish (optional)

1. Combine all of the ingredients, except the cilantro, in a slow cooker.

2. Cover and cook on high for 3 to 4 hours, or until the sweet potatoes are tender and the curry has thickened.

3. Divide the curry among bowls and garnish with chopped cilantro (if desired).

Per Serving: Calories: 245; Saturated Fat: 9g; Total Fat: 11g; Protein: 8g; Total Carbs: 30g; Fiber: 7g; Sodium: 275mg

BUENO BREAKFAST BURRITO

VEGAN Take control over what goes into your tortilla with this healthy, plant-protein-packed, energizing breakfast. You may be turned off by a tofu-stuffed burrito, but I dare you to try this recipe. It might just become a staple in your diet. Organic tofu is a great source of protein, iron, and calcium.

Yield: 6 servings
Prep: 20 minutes
Cook: 20 minutes

¾ cup roasted salted cashews
¾ cup mild chunky salsa
¼ cup nutritional yeast
¼ teaspoon onion powder
¼ teaspoon garlic powder
¼ teaspoon ground cumin
1 tablespoon canola oil
½ cup water or vegetable broth
14 ounces extra-firm tofu
Juice of 1 lime
Salt
6 large flour tortillas
2 tablespoons chopped fresh cilantro
1½ cups roasted potatoes, for serving (optional)

1. In a high-speed blender, combine the cashews, salsa, nutritional yeast, onion powder, garlic powder, cumin, canola oil, and water and blend until completely smooth.

2. Drain the tofu and pat dry.

3. Put the tofu in a large skillet over medium-high heat. Use a potato masher to mash the tofu until it resembles scrambled eggs.

4. Add the cashew sauce and lime juice, and season with salt.

5. Cook the tofu for about 15 minutes, or until the moisture begins to evaporate and it becomes a little less mushy.

6. Spoon the tofu mixture into the tortillas, add the chopped cilantro, and roll up the burritos.

7. Serve immediately, with roasted potatoes (if desired), or refrigerate or freeze for later.

Ingredient tip: You can find tofu at most grocery stores, either in the produce or vegan food refrigerated sections. Buy tofu made with organic, non-GMO soybeans. Firm and extra-firm tofu hold up well for cutting into cubes, whereas silken tofu is better for sauces, smoothies and baking. Open the package over the sink to drain the water in the package.

Per Serving: Calories: 434; Saturated Fat: 2g; Total Fat: 22g; Protein: 19g; Total Carbs: 43g; Fiber: 5g; Sodium: 686mg

16

CHAPTER

Recipes for Rest Days

GARLIC TAHINI DRESSING 154

EASY TENDER OVEN-BAKED CHICKEN 155

LAZY BEEF BOWL 156

MAPLE-DIJON–GLAZED SALMON 157

PINEAPPLE FRIED RICE 158

SESAME-HONEY TEMPEH WITH WILD RICE 159

SOUTHWESTERN SALAD 160

NO-BAKE CHOCOLATE PEANUT BUTTER
CELEBRATION TREATS 161

GARLIC TAHINI DRESSING

DAIRY-FREE, GLUTEN-FREE, VEGETARIAN Salads are packed with vitamins and minerals, but using a store-bought dressing often undoes those health benefits. Most bottled dressings are packed with artificial flavors, sodium, sugar, and oils. Making your own dressing puts you in charge of the ingredients, and it's far less expensive. This recipe's combination of tahini and garlic, with a touch of honey and lemon, is sure to please your taste buds.

Yield: 1 cup
Prep: 10 minutes

⅓ cup tahini

¼ cup freshly squeezed lemon juice

2 garlic cloves, minced

½ teaspoon salt

1 teaspoon honey

¼ to ⅓ cup water

1. In a food processor, combine the tahini, lemon juice, garlic, salt, and honey. Add ¼ cup of water and pulse 4 to 6 times, or until the dressing is smooth. Add more water as needed to meet your desired consistency.

2. Transfer to a leakproof salad dressing bottle or container and refrigerate until ready to use.

Storage: The dressing will keep in the refrigerator for up to 1 week.

Ingredient tip: Tahini is a ground sesame seed paste that's found in many Middle Eastern dishes. Since it has a very high oil content, be sure to thoroughly mix it before you refrigerate it. You can find tahini in most supermarkets; check the condiment aisle near specialty olives or the ethnic foods section.

Per Serving (1 tablespoon): Calories: 32; Saturated Fat: 0g; Total Fat: 3g; Protein: 1g; Total Carbs: 2g; Fiber: 2g; Sodium: 68mg

EASY TENDER OVEN-BAKED CHICKEN

DAIRY-FREE, GLUTEN-FREE, PALEO This recipe is truly a "winner, winner, chicken dinner." It's one of those quick and easy meals you'll find yourself repeating every week. The brine called for in this recipe makes the most juicy and tender meat. Aside from the chicken, you only need a few ingredients from your spice cabinet. Be sure to bake an extra batch on the weekend and use it in place of deli meat in your sandwich or on top of a salad.

Yield: 4 servings
Prep: 20 minutes
Cook: 25 minutes

4 boneless, skinless chicken breasts (about 2½ pounds)

4 cups warm water

3 tablespoons kosher salt, plus ½ teaspoon

⅓ teaspoon freshly ground black pepper

½ teaspoon garlic powder

½ teaspoon paprika

1 to 2 tablespoons olive oil

1. Depending on the thickness of your chicken breasts, either pound them out or slice them horizontally to create even cuts, about ¾ inch thick.

2. In a large bowl, combine the warm water with 3 tablespoons of kosher salt. Stir until most of the salt is dissolved.

3. Add the chicken breasts to the saltwater and let them brine for about 15 minutes.

4. While the chicken is brining, in a small bowl, combine the remaining ½ teaspoon of salt, pepper, garlic powder, and paprika and set aside.

5. Preheat the oven to 450°F.

6. Remove the chicken breasts from the brine, rinse with cold water, and pat dry with paper towels.

7. Place the chicken breasts in a single layer in a large baking dish. Brush both sides of the chicken with the olive oil, then sprinkle both sides evenly with the spice mixture.

8. Bake the chicken for 16 to 17 minutes, or until cooked through and no longer pink. Switch the oven to broil. Flip the chicken and broil for 3 minutes, or until lightly browned.

9. Remove the baking dish from the oven and cover loosely with aluminum foil. Let the chicken rest for 5 minutes before serving.

Ingredient tip: The labels natural, cage-free, farm-raised, and free-range don't necessarily mean that your chicken was pasture-raised. Look for the USDA organic label to ensure that your chicken was raised on entirely organic feed. This label also means that the chicken is free of antibiotics and hormones.

Per Serving: Calories: 120; Saturated Fat: 0g; Total Fat: 4g; Protein: 20g; Total Carbs: 0g; Fiber: 0g; Sodium: 183mg

LAZY BEEF BOWL

GLUTEN-FREE A mouthwatering beef bowl in less than 25 minutes? That's where the "lazy" comes in. The sirloin in this recipe is high in protein. Beef also contains a generous amount of B vitamins, selenium, zinc, and phosphorus, and is rich in heme iron. Boost the nutritional value of your bowl by serving the beef over cooked rice and steamed broccoli.

Yield: 4 servings
Prep: 10 minutes
Cook: 15 minutes

3 tablespoons packed brown sugar

¼ cup reduced-sodium soy sauce (or gluten-free tamari)

2 teaspoons sesame oil

¾ teaspoon grated peeled fresh ginger

2 dashes red pepper flakes

1 tablespoon canola oil

3 garlic cloves, minced

1 pound ground sirloin

2 scallions, thinly sliced

½ teaspoon sesame seeds

Crushed peanuts, for garnish (optional)

1. In a small bowl, whisk together the brown sugar, soy sauce, sesame oil, grated ginger, and red pepper flakes.

2. Heat the oil in a large skillet over medium to medium-high heat. Add the garlic, stirring constantly, until fragrant. Add the ground beef and cook, breaking up the meat with a wooden spoon, for 6 to 7 minutes. Drain any excess fat from the pan.

3. Stir the soy sauce mixture and scallions into the beef and cook until heated through.

4. Top with the sesame seeds and crushed peanuts (if using), and serve immediately.

Leftovers tip: Make extra and enjoy leftovers stuffed in a tortilla with chopped lettuce or cabbage, and your favorite dressing.

Per Serving: Calories: 279; Saturated Fat: 5g; Total Fat: 15g; Protein: 25g; Total Carbs: 8g; Fiber: 0g; Sodium: 588mg

MAPLE-DIJON–GLAZED SALMON

PALEO Tasty and versatile, salmon is one of the best sources of omega-3 fatty acids (which may help reduce muscle soreness and pain), EPA, and DHA. Commonly touted for its heart-health and brain-boosting benefits, this nutrient-packed power food should be in every athlete's meal rotation. This recipe is an excellent source of protein and will help you repair damaged muscles on your day off from exercise.

Yield: 3 servings
Prep: 10 minutes
Cook: 15 minutes

2 skin-on salmon fillets
(about 1 pound total)
Pinch salt
Freshly ground black pepper
2 tablespoons maple syrup
1 tablespoon Dijon mustard
(preferably whole-grain)
1 teaspoon apple cider vinegar
½ teaspoon Worcestershire
sauce
1 tablespoon olive oil, plus
more for greasing

1. Preheat the oven to 400°F. Line a baking sheet with aluminum foil and lightly oil it.

2. Sprinkle the salmon fillets with salt and pepper.

3. In a small bowl, whisk together the maple syrup, Dijon mustard, vinegar, Worcestershire sauce, and 1 tablespoon of olive oil.

4. Place the salmon fillets skin-side down on the prepared baking sheet and brush the top of the fish generously with the maple-Dijon glaze.

5. Bake the salmon for about 10 minutes (cooking time will vary depending on thickness of the fillets). Switch the oven to broil and broil the salmon for 1 to 2 minute to crisp up the top.

6. Serve the salmon with sides of your choice.

Ingredient tip: Farmed salmon is readily available, but given the questionable farming practices used around the world, I recommend wild-caught salmon. Look for wild-caught salmon that appears moist and vibrantly colored, with shades of red to bright pink. If fresh salmon is not available (or is out of your budget), choose frozen.

Per Serving: Calories: 303; Saturated Fat: 3g; Total Fat: 14g; Protein: 34g; Total Carbs: 9g; Fiber: 0g; Sodium: 350mg

PINEAPPLE FRIED RICE

DAIRY-FREE, GLUTEN-FREE, VEGETARIAN Rice is one of the world's leading food crops. Grown every continent except Antarctica, it's the staple food of more than half of the world's population. Rice is high in nutrients, vitamins, and minerals; low in fat; naturally sodium-free and an excellent source of fiber; plus it's versatile, inexpensive, and easy to make. I'm confident this Thai-inspired recipe will be one of your new weekly favorites. Be sure to complement this healthy, delicious and colorful dish with your favorite source of animal or plant protein.

Yield: 4 servings
Prep: 15 minutes
Cook: 35 minutes

1 cup long-grain brown rice

1¼ cups water

1½ tablespoons canola oil, divided

2 eggs, beaten

1½ cups chopped pineapple

1 red bell pepper, chopped

3 scallions, chopped

2 garlic cloves, minced

½ cup unsalted cashews, chopped

1 tablespoon reduced-sodium soy sauce (or gluten-free tamari)

2 teaspoons sweet chili sauce

1 lime, halved; one half cut into 4 wedges for garnish

Salt

Handful fresh cilantro leaves, chopped, for garnish

1. In a medium saucepan with a tight-fitting lid, combine the rice with the water. Bring to a boil over medium-high heat, then reduce the heat to low, cover, and cook for 30 minutes, or until all of the water is absorbed. Remove the pot from the heat, then fluff the rice with a fork. Let sit, covered, for 8 to 10 minutes.

2. Meanwhile, heat a large cast iron skillet or nonstick frying pan over medium heat. Put ½ teaspoon of oil in the pan and pour in the eggs. Stir the eggs frequently until scrambled and lightly set. Transfer the eggs to a bowl. Wipe out the pan if necessary.

3. Add 1 tablespoon of oil to the pan, then add the pineapple and red pepper. Stir frequently, until the red pepper is tender and the pineapple is caramelized on the edges. Add the scallions and garlic and cook until fragrant, continuing to stir.

4. Move the pineapple mixture to one side of the pan and add the remaining 1 teaspoon of oil to the other side of the pan. Add the chopped cashews to the oil side of the pan and cook until fragrant. Continue to stir.

5. Add the rice to the pan and stir everything to combine. Cook, stirring occasionally, until the rice is hot. Add the scrambled eggs, soy sauce, and chili sauce. Cook until warmed through.

6. Squeeze the juice of ½ lime over the dish and stir to combine. Season with salt to taste.

7. Divide the fried rice among plates and garnish each with a lime wedge and a sprinkle of cilantro.

Make-ahead tip: To save time, cook the rice ahead of time and keep it in an airtight container in the refrigerator. This will help prevent clumping in stir-fry dishes. The water-to-rice ratio can vary depending on the type of rice you use; for short-grain rice, use 1½ cups each water and rice.

Per Serving: Calories: 223; Saturated Fat: 2g; Total Fat: 11g; Protein: 6g; Total Carbs: 26g; Fiber: 2g; Sodium: 167mg

SESAME-HONEY TEMPEH WITH WILD RICE

DAIRY-FREE, GLUTEN-FREE, VEGETARIAN Tempeh is made from cooked whole soybeans that are fermented into a firm, dense patty. It's considered a staple in vegetarian and vegan diets. Although it looks a little strange in the package, this minimally processed food brings a nutty, chewy, and "meaty" flavor to dishes, and also does a great job of absorbing other flavors. Tempeh provides all the amino acids that your body needs, plus it has probiotic benefits derived from the fermentation process. This is an excellent dish to refuel your energy, boost your immune system, and speed muscle healing.

Yield: 4 servings
Prep: 10 minutes
Cook: 15 minutes

2 tablespoons sesame oil

3 tablespoons honey

2 tablespoons gluten-free tamari

2 tablespoons water

1 teaspoon cornstarch

2 (8-ounce) packages tempeh, crumbled into bite-size pieces

4 cups cooked wild rice

Leafy greens, for serving

Sliced scallions, for garnish

1. In a medium bowl, mix together the sesame oil, honey, tamari, water, and cornstarch.

2. Add the crumbled tempeh to the bowl and toss until evenly coated.

3. In a large nonstick skillet over medium heat, cook the tempeh mixture for 8 to 10 minutes, or until golden brown. Toss every few minutes to prevent burning.

4. For each serving, place ½ cup tempeh and 1 cup cooked wild rice over a bed of leafy greens. Garnish with scallions.

Ingredient tip: Look for tempeh in the refrigerated section of your grocery or natural food store, near the tofu or meat alternatives. Don't be put off by its appearance. Tempeh is a fermented soy product, so you may see a few black spots with white stuff in between. Technically, that is mold, but it's entirely normal and perfectly edible. (You can cut it off if you prefer.) If tempeh is slimy, sticky, or smells sour, however, throw it out. To make this recipe vegan, use apple honey instead of regular honey.

Per Serving: Calories: 502; Saturated Fat: 5g; Total Fat: 20g; Protein: 30g; Total Carbs: 58g; Fiber: 3g; Sodium: 524mg

SOUTHWESTERN SALAD

VEGETARIAN Eating a salad is one of the simplest and healthiest habits you can adopt. Salad is often the first thing that athletes turn to when they want to cut back on calories or boost nutritional intake, and a good one should also leave you feeling satisfied and energized. A traditional Southwestern salad is loaded with cheese and drenched in a creamy dressing, and it's sometimes served in a high-calorie fried tortilla bowl. This version is a healthy alternative, loaded with fiber and antioxidants, and full of flavor.

Yield: 2 servings
Prep: 15 minutes

FOR THE DRESSING:

¼ cup ranch dressing
    (homemade or bottled
    ranch yogurt dressing)

2 tablespoons light sour cream

½ teaspoon chili powder

½ teaspoon apple cider vinegar

½ teaspoon freshly
squeezed lime juice

¼ teaspoon ground cumin

3 dashes garlic powder

3 dashes onion powder

Dash hot sauce (optional, if
    you like a little extra spice)

FOR THE SALAD:

2 cups spinach, any large
    stems removed

4 cups lettuce, such as green
    leaf, red leaf, or a mix

½ cup canned black beans,
    drained and rinsed

½ cup canned corn, drained

½ cup thinly sliced carrots

2 tablespoons chopped
    fresh cilantro

2 tablespoons shredded
    Cheddar cheese (optional)

½ avocado, chopped (optional)

½ lime, cut into 4 wedges

12 tortilla chips

1. In a medium bowl, mix together all of the ingredients for the dressing.

2. Divide the salad ingredients and assemble on two large plates, starting with the spinach and lettuce, then topping with the beans, corn, carrots, cilantro, cheese, and avocado (if using).

3. Finish with a drizzle of dressing.

4. Serve each salad with 2 lime wedges and 6 tortilla chips. Squeeze lime juice over the salads and either crumble the tortilla chips over the salads or eat on the side.

Ingredient tip: For a protein boost, add grilled chicken, shrimp, beef, tofu, or a meatless burger.

Leftovers tip: If you have extra dressing, use it for dipping veggies, as a sandwich spread, or to top baked or roasted potatoes.

Per Serving (without dressing): Calories: 177; Saturated Fat: 2g; Total Fat: 6g; Protein: 9g; Total Carbs: 48g; Fiber: 8g; Sodium: 170mg

NO-BAKE CHOCOLATE PEANUT BUTTER CELEBRATION TREATS

VEGETARIAN All over the world, food is an important part of any celebration. Whether you're celebrating a team victory or a personal best, these no-bake treats are an excellent choice. Filled with delicious chocolate and peanut butter, they're sure to satisfy a sweet tooth. I suggest keeping only a few out at a time and freezing the rest. Trust me, they're irresistible!

Yield: About 4 dozen
Prep: 5 minutes
Cook: 10 minutes

2 cups sugar

½ cup unsalted butter

½ cup unsweetened cocoa

½ cup low-fat milk

1 cup peanut butter

1½ teaspoons vanilla extract

3 cups quick-cooking oats

1. In a saucepan over medium heat, combine the sugar, butter, cocoa, and milk. Bring to a quick boil, stirring constantly. Reduce the heat to medium and cook for 3 to 4 minutes, continuing to stir constantly.

2. Remove from the heat and stir in the peanut butter, vanilla, and oats.

3. Drop heaping teaspoonfuls of the mixture onto wax paper. Be sure to do this while the mixture is still warm because it will be more difficult as the mixture cools.

4. Let the treats cool on the wax paper until hardened.

Storage: Store the treats in an airtight container in the refrigerator until ready to eat. You can also freeze them in a heavy-duty freezer bag for up to 6 months.

Recipe tip: If you're too rigid, restrictive, or strict about food, that can cause problems. There's a fine line between carefully considering what goes into your body and excessively obsessing over every food calorie. If you have a healthy relationship with food, nothing, including these treats, should be off limits. It's okay to loosen the food rules sometimes. Remember, a balanced diet is not about perfection.

Per Serving: Calories: 102; Saturated Fat: 2g; Total Fat: 5g; Protein: 2g; Total Carbs: 13g; Fiber: 1g; Sodium: 26mg

GLOSSARY

A

Aerophagia Excessive and repetitive air swallowing.

Air-displacement plethysmography A method to determine body composition (fat vs. lean mass).

Aldosterone A steroid hormone produced in the adrenal glands.

Alpha-linolenic acid (ALA) Omega-3 fatty acid found in plant sources such as nuts and seeds.

Amenorrhea The absence (primary amenorrhea) or cessation (secondary amenorrhea) of normal menstrual function.

Amino acids Organic compounds that act as building blocks of proteins and play a role in metabolism.

Anabolic The building up of body tissue.

Anemia A lack of red blood cells or dysfunctional red blood cells in the body.

Antibiotics Strong medicines designed to fight infections by killing bacteria or keeping them from reproducing.

Antibodies A protective protein produced by the immune system in response to a foreign invader.

Antidiuretic hormone (ADH) A hormone made in the hypothalamus and stored in the pituitary. ADH helps the kidneys control the water quantity excreted in the urine.

Antioxidants A substance that may protect cells from free radical damage.

Arachidonic acid Polyunsaturated omega-6 fatty acid.

B

Beta-alanine Nonessential amino acid. When supplemented, may increase skeletal muscle carnosine concentrations to buffer and reduce acidity in active muscles.

Bicarbonate Electrolyte used by the body to help maintain the body's acid-base (pH) balance and to keep your body hydrated.

Bioelectrical impedance analysis (BIA) A method of measuring body fat in relation to lean body mass when assessing body composition.

Biological value (BV) A measurement of how well and rapidly your body can digest and absorb the protein you consume.

Blood volume (BV) The volume of blood in the circulatory system, specifically from red blood cells and plasma volume. Regulated by the kidneys, the typical adult blood volume is ~5 liters.

Branch chain amino acids (BCAAs) Specific essential amino acids—leucine, isoleucine, and valine—that play a role in metabolism, immunity and brain function.

C

Carbohydrates A large group of organic compounds containing hydrogen and oxygen that can be broken down to release energy in the body. Found in food and living tissues such as cellulose, sugars and starch.

Cardiac output (CO) The amount of blood pumped by the heart per minute. CO = heart rate × stroke volume.

Cardiovascular drift The natural increase in heart rate coupled with a decline in stroke volume that occurs during prolonged exercise, despite exercise intensity remaining the same.

Cholesterol A natural waxy, fat like substance made by the body and found in food. Needed to make hormones, vitamin D and digestive substances.

Creatine The liver, pancreas, and kidneys make creatine, and the body converts it to phosphocreatine, which is stored in the muscles for energy. Found in food or as a supplement.

Cryotherapy Cold therapy treatment involving the use of freezing or near-freezing temperatures.

D

Daily reference intakes (DRI) This general term provides a set of reference values to plan and assess nutrient intake. The four DRI's include the Recommended Dietary Allowance (RDA), Adequate Intake (AI), Tolerable Intake Level (UL) and Estimated Average Requirement (EAR).

Dehydration A condition when your body doesn't have as much water as it needs to function properly.

Delayed onset muscle soreness (DOMS) Muscle pain and stiffness that develops a day or two after a heavy bout of exercise.

Disaccharides A double sugar formed when two monosaccharides are joined together.

Docosahexaenoic acid (DHA) Polyunsaturated omega-3 fatty acid. A major structural fat found in the brain and eyes.

Dual-energy X-ray absorptiometry (DXA or DEXA) A method of measuring bone mineral density through two X-ray beams.

E

Eicosapentaenoic acid (EPA) Omega-3 fatty acid found in oily fish and seafood.

Electrolytes Substances that have the ability to conduct electricity. Present in the human body, their balance is critical for normal functioning of cells and organs.

Endothelium A thin layer of cells that line the inside surface of blood and lymphatic vessels.

Erythropoietin (EPO) A hormone secreted by the kidneys that stimulates red blood cell production in the bone marrow.

F

Fat Also known as triglycerides, fats are a necessary dietary component serving metabolic and structural functions.

Female athlete triad A female syndrome involving eating disorders (or low energy availability), amenorrhea/oligomenorrhea, and decreased bone mineral density (osteoporosis and osteopenia).

Fluid balance To keep body fluids within a healthy range in order to maintain homeostasis, the amount of water lost from the body must equal the amount taken.

Food and Drug Administration (FDA) Federal agency of the U.S. Department of Health and Human Services. Responsible for protecting and promoting public health.

Fructose A simple sugar also known as fruit sugar.

G

Galactose Naturally occurring monosaccharide found in milk and dairy products.

Gastric emptying The natural process when food, liquid, and digestive juice contents empty from the stomach and into the small intestine.

Gene The basic unit of heredity made up of DNA.

Gluconeogenesis A metabolic process used to create glucose from non-carbohydrate substances to keep blood glucose levels from dropping too low.

Glucose A simple sugar food source that is an important energy source for the brain and muscles. Also known as blood sugar.

Glycemic index (GI) A value assigned to foods based on how slowly or quickly they increase blood glucose levels.

Glycemic load (GL) A number that estimates the carbohydrate quantity in a portion of food relative to how quickly it raises blood glucose levels.

Glycogen A multibranched polysaccharide that serves as the main storage form of glucose in the human body.

H

Heat cramps Painful, involuntary muscle spasms that typically occur during heavy exercise in very warm environments.

Heat exhaustion A heat-related illness that results in the body overheating.

Heatstroke A heat-related illness when the body's temperature-regulating mechanism fails when exposed to excessively high temperatures.

Homeostasis A state of stable equilibrium.

Hydrostatic weighing Underwater mechanism for measuring body fat percentage.

Hypertonic A solution that has more solute and less water.

Hypotonic A solution that has less solute and more water.

Hyponatremia A high concentration of sodium in the blood (>145 mmol/L).

L

Lactose A disaccharide containing glucose and galactose. Present in milk.

Lean body mass Component of body composition not from fat.

Leucine Essential amino acid used in protein synthesis and metabolic functioning.

Linoleic acid Polyunsaturated omega-3 fatty acid found mostly in plant oils.

M

Macronutrients The type of food (carbohydrates, protein, fat) required in large amounts in the diet.

Maltose A disaccharide sugar produced by the breakdown of starch.

Menopause A natural decline in reproductive hormones when a woman's ovaries stop producing estrogen and progesterone.

Micronutrients Essential elements needed in small quantities (generally less than 100 mg a day) to maintain health.

Minerals Chemical elements required to perform functions necessary for life. The five major minerals in the human body are calcium, sodium, potassium, magnesium, and phosphorous.

Monosaccharides The simplest forms of carbohydrates, which include glucose, fructose, and galactose.

Monounsaturated fats Commonly found in plant foods, these are liquid at room temperature. Often called the "good" fat.

N

Nonsteroidal anti-inflammatory drugs (NSAIDs) They block enzymes that play a role in making prostaglandins, which means less pain and swelling.

O

Omega-3 fatty acids A class of essential polyunsaturated fatty acids with the initial double bond in the third carbon position from the methyl terminal.

Omega-6 fatty acids A class of essential polyunsaturated fatty acids with the initial double bond in the sixth carbon position from the methyl group.

Omnivore A person who consumes food from plant and animal sources.

Osmolality A measure of the quantity of dissolved particles in a fluid.

Osmosis To equalize the concentration of solute on two sides of a membrane, this describes the movement of a solvent through a semipermeable membrane into a higher solute concentration.

Osteoporosis Also known as porous bone, this describes a bone disease when the body makes too little bone or loses too much bone, or both. Bones can become weak and may break.

P

Phytoestrogens Dietary estrogens that naturally occur in plants.

Polyphenols Naturally occurring micronutrients found largely in fruits, vegetables, cereals, and beverages that may have health benefits when consumed.

Polysaccharides Carbohydrates (i.e., glycogen, cellulose, starch) whose molecules consist of long chains of monosaccharide units bonded together by glycosidic linkages.

Polyunsaturated fats Healthy fats that contain more than one unsaturated carbon bond. Found in plant and animal foods.

Prebiotics Natural, non-digestible food components that promote the growth of healthy bacteria in the gut.

Probiotics Naturally found in your gut, food or supplements, these live and active cultures help change and repopulate intestinal bacteria to optimize gut flora.

Protein A macronutrient which plays many critical roles in the body. Built from building blocks called amino acids.

Protein digestibility–corrected amino acid score (PDCAAS) A measurement that uses the digestibility of a food protein and an amino acid profile. The result describes the protein's ability to provide adequate levels of essential amino acids for human needs.

R

Relative energy deficiency in sport (RED-S) The result of insufficient caloric intake and/or excessive energy expenditure. Adapted from the female athlete triad.

Resting metabolic rate (RMR) The rate at which your body burns calories when it is at complete rest.

S

Saturated fats Fats that do not have double bonds between carbon molecules because they are saturated with hydrogen molecules. Typically solid at room temperature.

Starch Complex carbohydrate consisting of many glucose units joined by glycosidic bonds.

Stroke volume The volume of blood pumped from the left ventricle of the heart in one contraction.

Sucrose Disaccharide made of half glucose and half fructose. Main component of cane or beet sugar.

T

Testosterone A steroid hormone produced primarily in the testicles that helps maintain bone density, muscle mass, body hair, sex drive and sperm production. Also produced in the ovaries and adrenal cortex.

Triglycerides A type of fat (lipid) found in the blood to provide energy. Excess calories are turned into triglycerides and stored in fat cells. High levels may contribute to thickening of the artery walls, which increases risk of stroke, heart attack and heart disease.

U

Unsaturated fats Fatty acids or fats with at least one double bond within the fatty acid chain. Can be mono (one) or poly (more than one).

Urine specific gravity The concentration of waste molecules excreted from the urine. The normal adult range is 1.01 to 1.03.

U.S. Department of Agriculture (USDA) Federal department responsible for developing and executing laws related to farming, forestry, and food.

V

Visceral fat Excess abdominal fat stored deep underneath the skin that may wrap around major organs, such as the liver, pancreas, and intestines. In excess, the risk for heart attacks, type 2 diabetes, cancer and stroke increases.

Vitamins Organic water or fat-soluble compounds needed in small quantities to support life. Vitamin consumption should come primarily from food.

RESOURCES

Academy of Nutrition and Dietetics: www.eatright.org
Your go-to source for science-based food and nutrition information.

Informed-Sport: www.informed-sport.com/
The best website to learn about supplements that have undergone a rigorous certification process.

International Society of Sports Nutrition: www.sportsnutritionsociety.org
The only non-profit academic society dedicated to promoting the science and application of evidence-based sports nutrition and supplementation, providing the most trusted resource in the world of sports supplements and nutrition—the peer-reviewed Medline indexed journal (www.jissn.com).

Medline Plus: www.medlineplus.gov/
Produced by the National Library of Medicine, this website provides up-to-date information about diseases, health conditions, and wellness issues in easy-to-understand language.

National Eating Disorders Association: www.nationaleatingdisorders.org
This is the website for the largest nonprofit organization dedicated to supporting individuals and families affected by eating disorders. Check it out for information on prevention, cures, and access to quality care.

Nutrition.gov: www.nutrition.gov
This USDA-sponsored website is a credible source of information to help you make healthy eating choices.

Sports, Cardiovascular, and Wellness Nutrition (SCAN): www.scandpg.org
The largest dietetic practice group of the Academy of Nutrition and Dietetics, dedicated to nutrition for sports performance and physical activity, cardiovascular health, wellness and eating disorders, and disordered eating.

Supplement 411: www.usada.org/substances/supplement-411/
Check out this site to get better informed about high-risk supplements so you can reduce your risk of testing positive for a banned substance or experiencing adverse health effects.

World Anti-Doping Agency: www.wada-ama.org/
This website is for athletes, coaches, parents, and anyone else who wants to learn more about anti-doping rules and regulations.

REFERENCES

"A Brief History of USDA Food Guides." United States Department of Agriculture. Accessed May 7, 2018. https://www.choosemyplate.gov/brief-history-usda-food-guides.

"Allergies." Mayo Clinic. Accessed June 1, 2018. https://www.mayoclinic.org/diseases-conditions/allergies/symptoms-causes/syc-20351497.

"Asthma." Mayo Clinic. Accessed June 1, 2018. https://www.mayoclinic.org/diseases-conditions/asthma/symptoms-causes/syc-20369653.

"Basic Information About Your Drinking Water." United States Environmental Protection Agency, 2018. Accessed May 1, 2018. https://www.epa.gov/ground-water-and-drinking-water/basic-information-about-your-drinking-water.

Brouns, Fred, and Ed Beckers. "Is the Gut an Athletic Organ?" *Sports Medicine* 15, no. 4 (1993): 242-257.

Buettner, Dan. "Why Japan's Longest-Lived Women Hold the Key to Better Health." *Huffington Post*. Last modified December 6, 2017. https://www.huffingtonpost.com/dan-buettner/okinawa-blue-zone_b_7012042.html.

Byrne, Shannon, Danielle Barry, and Nancy M. Petry. "Predictors of Weight Loss Success. Exercise Vs. Dietary Self-Efficacy and Treatment Attendance." *Appetite* 58, no. 2 (2012): 695-698 doi:10.1016/j.appet.2012.01.005.

Caspero, Alexandra. "Protein and the Athlete—How Much Do You Need?" *EatRight*. July 17, 2017. https://www.eatright.org/fitness/sports-and-performance/fueling-your-workout/protein-and-the-athlete.

Cengiz, Asim, and Bilal Demirhan. "Physiology of Wrestlers' Dehydration." *Turkish Journal of Sport and Exercise* 15, no. 2 (2013): 1-10 https://pdfs.semanticscholar.org/869c/a9036906b0b9eb47c7da98f45576c279adfc.pdf.

Chambers, Ashley, and Len Kravitz. "Nutrient Timing: The New Frontier in Fitness Performance." *UNM.edu*. Accessed May 22, 2018. https://www.unm.edu/~lkravitz/Article%20folder/nutrientUNM.html.

Clark, Nancy. "Nutrition Support Programs for Young Adult Athletes." *International Journal of Sport Nutrition* 8, no. 4 (1998): 416-425. doi:10.1123/ijsn.8.4.416.

Collier, R. "Intermittent Fasting: The Science of Going Without." *Canadian Medical Association Journal* 185, no. 9 (2013): E363-E364. doi:10.1503/cmaj.109-4451.

Cymerman, Allen. "Nutritional Needs in Cold and in High-Altitude Environments: Applications for Military Personnel in Field Operations." Institute of Medicine (US) Committee on Military Nutrition Research, 1996. Accessed May 26, 2018. https://www.ncbi.nlm.nih.gov/books/NBK232874/.

Daroux-Cole, L, R. Pettengell, and A. Jewell. "Exercise for Cancer Survivors: A Review." *OA Cancer* 1, no. 1 (2013) http://www.oapublishinglondon.com/article/544.

"Dietary Reference Intakes: Water, Potassium, Sodium, Chloride, and Sulfate." *Institute of Medicine of the National Academies,* February 11, 2004. http://www.nationalacademies.org/hmd/Reports/2004/Dietary-Reference-Intakes-Water-Potassium-Sodium-Chloride-and-Sulfate.aspx.

"Feeding Your Child Athlete." *KidsHealth from Nemours.* Accessed May 12, 2018. http://kidshealth.org/en/parents/feed-child-athlete.html.

Fenichel, Patrick, Nicolas Chevalier, and Francoise Brucker-Davis. "Bisphenol A: An Endocrine and Metabolic Disruptor." *Annales D'endocrinologie* 74, no 3. (2013): 211-220. doi:10.1016/j.ando.2013.04.002.

"Football Player Body Composition: Importance of Monitoring for Performance and Health." Gatorade Sports Science Institute. Accessed May 27, 2018. http://www.gssiweb.org/sports-science-exchange/article/sse-145-football-player-body-composition-importance-of-monitoring-for-performance-and-health.

Gabel, Kathe A. "Special Nutritional Concerns for the Female Athlete." *Current Sports Medicine Reports* 5, no. 4 (2006): 187-191. doi:10.1097/01.CSMR.0000306505.78729.fb.

"Gender and Nutrition Issue Paper—Draft." Food and Agriculture Organization of the United Nations. October 2012. Accessed May 27, 2018. http://www.eldis.org/document/A63247.

German, J. Bruce, Angela M. Zivkovi, David C. Dallas, and Jennifer T. Smilowitz. "Nutrigenomics and Personalized Diets: What Will They Mean for Food?" *Annual Review of Food Science and Technology* 2, no. 1 (2011): 97-123. doi:10.1146/annurev.food.102308.124147.

Gleeson, Michael. "Immune Function and Exercise." *European Journal of Sport Science* 4, no. 3 (2004): 52-66. doi:10.1080/17461390400074304.

"Glycemic Index for 60+ Foods." Harvard Health Publishing. Last modified March 14, 2018. https://www.health.harvard.edu/diseases-and-conditions/glycemic-index-and-glycemic-load-for-100-foods.

Goertz, Sherry. "Gauging Fluid Balance with Osmolality." *Nursing* 36, no. 10 (October 2006): 70.

Gulati, Sonia. "The Role of Electrolytes in the Body." *SymptomFind.com.* May 7, 2016. https://www.symptomfind.com/nutrition-supplements/role-of-electrolytes-in-the-body/.

Hess, Julie, and Joanne Slavin. "Defining 'Protein' Foods." *Nutrition Today* 51, no. 3 (2016): 117-120. doi:10.1097/NT.0000000000000157.

"Heat-Related Illnesses (Heat Cramps, Heat Exhaustion, Heat Stroke)." Johns Hopkins Medicine. Accessed April 20, 2018. https://www.hopkinsmedicine.org/healthlibrary/conditions/pediatrics/heat-related_illnesses_heat_cramps_heat_exhaustion_heat_stroke_90,P01611.

Hoch, Anne Z., et al. "Is There an Association Between Athletic Amenorrhea and Endothelial Cell Dysfunction?" *Medicine and Science in Sports and Exercise* 35, no. 3 (2003): 377-383. doi:10.1249/01.MSS.0000053661.27992.75.

Holzman, David C. "Organic Food Conclusions Don't Tell the Whole Story." *Environmental Health Perspectives* 120, no. 12 (2012): a458. doi:10.1289/ehp.120-a458.

Hull, Michael V., et al. "Gender Differences and Access to a Sports Dietitian Influence Dietary Habits of Collegiate Athletes." *Journal of the International Society of Sports Nutrition* 13, no. 1 (2016). doi:10.1186/s12970-016-0149-4.

Huskisson, E., S. Maggini, and M. Ruf. "The Role of Vitamins and Minerals in Energy Metabolism and Well-Being." *Journal of International Medical Research* 35, no. 3 (2007): 277-289. doi:10.1177/147323000703500301.

"Hydration." Korey Stringer Institute, 2018. Accessed April 24, 2018. https://ksi.uconn.edu/prevention/hydration/.

"In a Thirsty World, Bottled Water Seems Wasteful." The Water Project. Accessed April 30, 2018. https://thewaterproject.org/bottled-water/bottled_water_wasteful.

Jeukendrup, Asker E., and Sophie C. Killer. "The Myths Surrounding Pre-Exercise Carbohydrate Feeding." *Annals of Nutrition and Metabolism* 57, no. 2 (2010): 18-25. doi:10.1159/000322698.

Karpinski, Christine, and Christine A. Rosenbloom. *Sports Nutrition: A Handbook for Professionals.* 6th ed. Chicago: Academy of Nutrition and Dietetics, 2017.

LaRosa, John. "Top 6 Trends for the Weight Loss Industry in 2018." *MarketResearch.com.* Accessed May 25, 2018. https://blog.marketresearch.com/top-6-trends-for-the-weight-loss-market-in-2018.

Leiper, John B. "Fate of Ingested Fluids: Factors Affecting Gastric Emptying and Intestinal Absorption of Beverages in Humans." *Nutrition Reviews* 73, no. 2 (2015): 57-72. doi:10.1093/nutrit/nuv032.

Lim, Allen. "Hydration and Nutrition for Endurance Athletes." YouTube video, 1:15:40. Peaks Coaching Group. May 26, 2015. https://www.youtube.com/watch?v=ZDHhNVt8jAE&t=1876s.

Lowery, Lonnie M. "Dietary Fat and Sports Nutrition: A Primer." *Journal of Sports Science and Medicine* 3, no. 3 (2014): 106-117.

Manore, Melinda M. "Weight Management for Athletes and Active Individuals: A Brief Review." *Sports Medicine* 45, no 1 (2015): 83-92. doi:10.1007/s40279-015-0401-0.

Maughan, R.J., J. Fallah, and E.F. Coyle. "The Effects of Fasting on Metabolism and Performance." *British Journal of Sports Medicine* 44, no. 7 (2010): 490-494. doi:10.1136/bjsm.2010.072181.

Maughan, Ronald J., et al. "IOC Consensus Statement: Dietary Supplements and the High-Performance Athlete." *British Journal of Sports Medicine* 52, no. 7 (2018): 439-455. doi:10.1136/bjsports-2018-099027.

McArdle, William D., Frank I. Katch, and Victor L. Katch. *Sports & Exercise Nutrition.* Philadelphia, PA: Lippincott Williams & Wilkins, 2018.

"Meeting Maternal Nutrition Needs During Lactation," from *Nutrition During Lactation.* Institute of Medicine (US) Committee on Nutritional Status During Pregnancy and Lactation. 1991. Accessed May 24, 2018. https://www.ncbi.nlm.nih.gov/books/NBK235579/.

Merry, Troy L., and Michael Ristow. "Do Antioxidant Supplements Interfere with Skeletal Muscle Adaptation to Exercise Training?" *The Journal of Physiology* 594, no. 18 (2016): 5135-5147. doi:10.1113/JP270654.

Mohebi-Nejad, Azin, and Behnood Bikdeli. "Omega-3 Supplements and Cardiovascular Diseases." *Tanaffos* 13, no. 1 (2014): 6-14.

Mountjoy, Margo, et al. "The IOC Consensus Statement: Beyond the Female Athlete Triad—Relative Energy Deficiency in Sport (RED-S)." *British Journal of Sports Medicine* 48, no. 7 (2014): 491-497. doi:10.1136/bjsports-2014-093502.

Myles, Ian A. "Fast Food Fever: Reviewing the Impacts of the Western Diet on Immunity." *Nutrition Journal* 13, no. 1 (2014): 13-61. doi:10.1186/1475-2891-13-61.

Murray, Bob. "How Curiosity Killed the Cramp: Emerging Science on the Cause and Prevention of Exercise-Associated Muscle Cramps." *Journal of the American Medical Athletic Association* 29, no. 3 (2016): 5-7.

Neubauer, Oliver, and Christina Yfanti. "Antioxidants in Athlete's Basic Nutrition." In *Antioxidants in Sport Nutrition*, edited by Manfred Lamprecht. Boca Raton, FL: CRC Press/Taylor & Francis, 2015.

Nichols, Andrew W. "Probiotics and Athletic Performance." *Current Sports Medicine Reports* 6, no. 4 (2007): 269-273.

Nisevich, Pamela A. "Sports Nutrition for Young Athletes: Vital to Victory." *Today's Dietitian* 10, no. 3 (2008): 44. http://www.todaysdietitian.com/newarchives/tdmarch2008pg44.shtml.

"Nutrition for the Traveling Athlete." Sports Dietitians Australia. Accessed May 13, 2018. https://www.sportsdietitians.com.au/factsheets/fuelling-recovery/nutrition-for-the-travelling-athlete/.

O'Conner, Deborah L., et al. "Canadian Consensus on Female Nutrition: Adolescence, Reproduction, Menopause, and Beyond." *Journal of Obstetrics and Gynecology Canada* 38, no. 6 (2016): 508-554. doi:10.1016/j.jogc.2016.01.001.

Ormsbee, Michael, Christopher Bach, and Daniel Baur. "Pre-Exercise Nutrition: The Role of Macronutrients, Modified Starches and Supplements on Metabolism and Endurance Performance." *Nutrients* 6, no. 5 (2014): 1782-1808. doi:10.3390/nu6051782.

Paoli, Antonio. "Ketogenic Diet for Obesity: Friend or Foe?" *International Journal of Environmental Research and Public Health* 11, no. 2 (2014): 2092-2107. doi:10.3390/ijerph110202092.

Popkin, Barry M., Kristen E. D'Anci, and Irwin H. Rosenberg. "Water, Hydration and Health." *Nutrition Reviews* 68, no. 8 (2010): 439-458. doi:10.1111/j.1753-4887.2010.00304.x.

Reilly, T., J. Waterhouse, L.M. Burke, and J.M. Alonso. "Nutrition for Travel." *Journal of Sports Sciences* 25, no. 1 (2007): S125-S134. doi:10.1080/02640410701607445.

Reilly, T., G. Atkinson, and J. Waterhouse. "Travel Fatigue and Jet-Lag." *Journal of Sports Sciences* 15, no. 3 (1997): 365-369. doi:10.1080/026404197367371.

Robinson, Justin. "What You Need to Know About Nutrient Timing." *AceFitness.org.* Accessed May 22, 2018. https://www.acefitness.org/education-and-resources/professional/expert-articles/5815/what-you-need-to-know-about-nutrient-timing.

Rogerson, David. "Vegan Diets: Practical Advice for Athletes and Exercisers." *Journal of the International Society of Sports Nutrition* 14, no. 1 (2017). doi:10.1186/s12970-017-0192-9.

Rolls, Barbara J., Ingrid C. Fedoroff, and Joanne F. Guthrie. "Gender Differences in Eating Behavior and Body Weight Regulation." *Health Psychology* 10, no. 2 (1991): 133-142.

Ronsen, Ola. "Nutritional and Fluid Intake in Cross Country Skiing." In *Handbook of Sports Medicine and Science, Cross Country Skiing*, edited by Heikki Rusko. John Wiley & Sons, 2008. doi:10.1080/02640414.2011.574721.

Rosenbloom, Christine A., and Ellen J. Coleman. *Sport Nutrition: A Handbook for Professionals.* 5th ed. Chicago: Academy of Nutrition and Dietetics, 2012.

Shmerling, Robert H. "The Latest Scoop on the Health Benefits of Coffee " *Harvard Health Blog.* September 25, 2017. https://www.health.harvard.edu/blog/the-latest-scoop-on-the-health-benefits-of-coffee-2017092512429.

Slater, Gary, and Stuart M. Phillips. "Nutrition Guidelines for Strength Sports: Sprinting, Weightlifting, Throwing Events, and Bodybuilding." *Journal of Sports Sciences* 29, no. 1 (2011): S67-S77. doi:10.1080/02640414.2011.574722.

Stanhope, Kimber L. "Sugar Consumption, Metabolic Disease and Obesity: The State of the Controversy." *Critical Reviews in Clinical Laboratory Sciences* 53, no. 1 (2015): 52-67. doi:10.3109/10408363.2015.1084990.

Tarnopolsky, M.A. "Gender Differences in Metabolism: Nutrition and Supplements." *Journal of Science and Sports Medicine* 3, no. 3 (2000): 287-298.

Taylor, Jennifer P., Susan Evers, and Mary McKenna. "Determinants of Healthy Eating in Children and Youth". *Canadian Journal of Public Health* 96, no. 3 (2005): S20-S26.

"The Athlete's Nutrition Needs." Nestlé. Accessed April 23, 2018. https://www.nestle.com.au/nhw/sports-nutrition/the-athletes-nutrition-needs.

"The Heath Benefits of Tea." *EatRight.* Accessed May 4, 2018. https://www.eatright.org/health/wellness/preventing-illness/the-health-benefits-of-tea.

Trexler, Eric T., Abbie E. Smith-Ryan, and Layne E. Norton. "Metabolic Adaptation to Weight Loss: Implications for the Athlete." *Journal of the International Society of Sports Nutrition* 11, no. 1 (2014). doi:10.1186/1550-2783-11-7.

Turocy, Paula Sammarone, et al. "National Athletic Trainers' Association Position Statement: Safe Weight Loss and Maintenance Practices in Sport and Exercise." *Journal of Athletic Training* 46, no. 3 (2011): 322-336.

Van Swearingen, Jessie M. "Nutrition and the Growing Athlete." *Journal of Orthopaedic and Sports Physical Therapy* 6, no. 3 (1984): 173-177.

Velayutham, Pon, Anandh Babu, and Dongmin, Liu. "Green Tea Catechins and Cardiovascular Health: An Update." *Current Medicinal Chemistry* 15, no. 18 (2008): 1840-1850.

Vella, Luke D., and David Cameron-Smith. "Alcohol, Athletic Performance and Recovery." *Nutrients* 2, no. 8 (2010): 781-789. doi:10.3390/nu2080781.

Venables, Michelle C., Juul Achten, and Asker E. Jeukendrup. "Determinants of Fat Oxidation During Exercise in Healthy Men and Women: A Cross-Sectional Study." *Journal of Applied Physiology* 98, no 1. (2005): 160-167. doi:10.1152/japplphysiol.00662.2003.

Wijnen, Annemarthe H.C., et al. "Post-Exercise Rehydration: Effect of Consumption of Beer with Varying Alcohol Content on Fluid Balance After Mild Dehydration." *Frontiers in Nutrition* 3, no. 45 (2016). doi:10.3389/fnut.2016.00045.

Wilmore, Jack H., and David L. Costill. *Physiology of Sport and Exercise*. 2nd ed. Champaign, IL: Human Kinetics, 1994.

INDEX

A

Aerophagia, 122
Age considerations, 91–92
Air-displacement
    plethysmography, 116
Alcohol, 36, 76, 104
Allergies, 127
Almond butter
    Almond Butter and Apple
        Sandwiches, 145
Altitude, 93
Amenorrhea, 96
Amino acids, 12, 18
Anemia, 86
Antibiotics, 125
Antioxidants, 28, 87
Apples
    Almond Butter and Apple
        Sandwiches, 145
Apricots, dried
    Apricot-Coconut
        Granola, 136
Asthma, 127
Autoimmune diseases, 128

B

Basketball, 112
Beef
    Lazy Beef Bowl, 156
Bell peppers
    Pineapple Fried Rice, 158
Berries
    Baked Blueberry
        Oatmeal, 137
    Berry-Cherry Smoothie, 148
    Blueberry-Stuffed Challah
        French Toast, 138
    Cinnamon Quinoa
        Bowl, 140
Bioelectrical impedance
    analysis, 116

Biological value (BV), 21
Black beans
    Southwestern Salad, 160
Blood volume, 31
Bodybuilding, 110
Body cavity fluid, 5
Body composition, 116. *See
    also* Weight
Body fat, 91, 92
Body image, men and, 95
Branch chain amino acids
    (BCAAs), 18, 86
Broccoli
    Slow Cooker Sweet Potato
        Quinoa Curry, 151

C

Caffeine, 34, 75, 87
Calcium, 4–5, 26, 86
Calories, 13
Cancer, 129
Carbohydrates
    complex, 15
    foundation diet
        planning, 41
    glycemic index (GI), 15–17
    overview, 2, 12, 13
    pre-workout
        recommendations,
        55–58
    simple, 13–14
    in sports drinks, 62–63
    storage of, 52–53
    workout recommendations,
        17, 66–67
Carbonated water, 32
Cardiovascular drift, 11
Carrots
    Carrot Cake Muffins, 139
    Southwestern Salad, 160
Casein, 19–20

Cheese. *See also* Cottage cheese
    Crust-Free Spinach,
        Mushroom, and Cheese
        Quiche, 150
    Organic Chickpea Fusilli
        with Goat Cheese, 149
    Over-Easy Grits Bowl, 141
    Southwestern Salad, 160
Cherries
    Apricot-Coconut
        Granola, 136
    Berry-Cherry Smoothie, 148
Chicken
    Easy Tender Oven-Baked
        Chicken, 155
Chickpeas
    Slow Cooker Sweet Potato
        Quinoa Curry, 151
Children, 100–105
Chloride, 4–5
Chocolate
    No-Bake Chocolate Peanut
        Butter Celebration
        Treats, 161
Chronic health issues, 126–129
Clock concentration, 132
Coconut
    Almond Butter and Apple
        Sandwiches, 145
    Apricot-Coconut
        Granola, 136
Coffee, 33–34, 124
Cold weather, 93
Competing. *See also*
        Pre-competition recipes
    children and student
        athletes, 102–103
    fluids while, 64–65
    foods while, 69–71
    post-competition
        fluids, 65–66

Competing. (*Continued*)
post-competition
food, 71–73
pre-competition
fluids, 54–55
pre-competition
foods, 58–60
rest days fluids, 76
rest days foods, 77–80
Concentration, 132
Corn
Southwestern Salad, 160
Cottage cheese
Sweet Potato Protein
Pancakes, 142
CrossFit, 110
Curcumin, 87–88
Cycling, distance, 108–109

D

Daily reference intake (DRI), 20
Dairy-free diets
Almond Butter and Apple
Sandwiches, 145
Baked Blueberry
Oatmeal, 137
Carrot Cake Muffins, 139
Easy Tender Oven-Baked
Chicken, 155
Garlic Tahini Dressing, 154
Peanut Butter Pretzel
Balls, 146
Perfect Pumpkin Energy
Balls, 147
Pineapple Fried Rice, 158
Sesame-Honey Tempeh with
Wild Rice, 159
Slow Cooker Sweet Potato
Quinoa Curry, 151
Dates
Peanut Butter Protein
Balls, 144
Perfect Pumpkin Energy
Balls, 147
Dehydration, 6–8, 9, 11,
30–31, 93

Delayed onset muscle soreness
(DOMS), 72, 124
Diabetes, 128–129
Diet. *See also* Nutrient timing;
Nutrition planning
children, 100–103
dining out, 43
foundational nutrition
planning, 38–42
hydration, 30–36
overview, 22, 37–38
special diets, 22, 43–49
Dining out, 43
Disaccharides, 14
Doping, 88
Drug use, 103–104
Dual-energy X-ray
absorptiometry
(DXA/DEXA), 116

E

Eating disorders
in student athletes, 105
in women, 98–99
Electrolytes, 4–6, 62
Endurance sports,
107–109
Energy drinks, 36
Erythropoietin (EPO), 88
Extracellular fluid, 5

F

Fasting, 56. *See also*
Intermittent fasting
Fats
foundation diet
planning, 42
omega-3 and omega-6 fatty
acids, 24
overview, 2, 12, 20–21
recommendations, 23
saturated, 21–22
unsaturated, 22–23
Female athlete triad, 96
Fermented foods, 37
Fiber, 15

Field events, 110
Figure skating, 114
Fluid(s)
absorption, 10
balance, 9
competition
recommendations, 64–65
dehydration, 6–8, 30–31
foundation diet planning, 41
intake, 9–10
loss, 8
overview, 4–6
post-workout
recommendations, 64
pre-competition
recommendations, 54–55
pre-workout
recommendations, 53–54
-related issues, 10–12
rest days recommendations,
75–76
types of, 31–36
workout recommendations,
62–63
FODMAPS diets, 48–49
Follicular phase, of
menstruation, 97
Football, 112
Fructose, 14
Fruits, 40, 75

G

Galactose, 14
Gastric emptying, 10
Gastro-intestinal (GI) issues,
15, 48, 56, 58, 122–123
Glucose, 13–14
Gluten-free diets, 46–47
Almond Butter and Apple
Sandwiches, 145
Cinnamon Quinoa Bowl, 140
Crust-Free Spinach,
Mushroom, and Cheese
Quiche, 150
Easy Tender Oven-Baked
Chicken, 155

Garlic Tahini Dressing, 154
Lazy Beef Bowl, 156
Organic Chickpea Fusilli
    with Goat Cheese, 149
Over-Easy Grits Bowl, 141
Peanut Butter Protein
    Balls, 144
Pineapple Fried Rice, 158
Sesame-Honey Tempeh with
    Wild Rice, 159
Slow Cooker Sweet Potato
    Quinoa Curry, 151
Sweet Potato Protein
    Pancakes, 142
Glycemic index (GI), 15–17
Glycemic load (GL), 16
Glycogen, 7, 15, 52, 79
Grains. *See* Whole grains
Grits
    Over-Easy Grits Bowl, 141
Gut health, 125. *See also*
        Gastro-intestinal
        (GI) issues
Gymnastics, 113

H

Heat-related issues, 11
High-intensity sports,
    112–114
Homeostasis, 4–6
Hormones, 91, 97, 98
Hydration. *See also*
        Dehydration; Fluid(s)
    children, 102
    overview, 4–6, 30
    and sweat, 7–8, 54
    and urine color, 7, 54, 76
Hyponatremia, 7, 12

I

Immune function, 124–126
Inflammation, 121
Injuries, 123
Insulin, 50
Intermittent fasting, 49
Intracellular fluid, 5

Iron, 19, 27, 86
Ironman triathlon, 107

J

Juice, 35–36

K

Ketogenic diets, 22, 47–48

L

Lactose, 14
Lean body mass, 92
Lettuce
    Southwestern Salad, 160
Leucine, 20, 82
Lifestyle factors, 125–126
Luteal phase, of menstru-
        ation, 97

M

Macronutrients, 23. *See also*
        Carbohydrates; Fats;
        Proteins
Magnesium, 4–5, 27
Maltose, 14
Marathons, 108
Meals. *See also*
        Post-workout recipes;
        Pre-competition recipes;
        Pre-workout recipes
    post-competition, 71–72
    post-workout, 68
    pre-competition, 59
    pre-workout, 56–57
    rest days, 77–78, 79–80
Men, 91, 95
Menopause, 98
Menstruation, 97
Mental health, men and, 95
Mental training, 130–133
Micronutrients, 23–24. *See also*
        Minerals; Vitamins
Milk, 34–35, 75
Mindfulness, 133
Minerals, 2, 23–24, 26–28
Monosaccharides, 13–14

Monounsaturated fats, 22
Muscle soreness, 72, 124
Mushrooms
    Crust-Free Spinach,
        Mushroom, and Cheese
        Quiche, 150
    Organic Chickpea Fusilli
        with Goat Cheese, 149

N

Negative self-talk, 131
Nonsteroidal
        anti-inflammatory drugs
        (NSAIDs), 121
Nordic skiing, 108
Nutrients
    carbohydrates, 13–17
    fats, 20–23, 24
    fluids and electrolytes, 4–12
    proteins, 18–20, 21
    sources of, 1–3, 12–13
    vitamins and minerals,
        23–28
Nutrient timing
    during competition,
        64–65, 69–71
    during exercise,
        62–63, 66–67
    overview, 50, 52–53
    post-competition,
        65–66, 71–73
    post-exercise, 64, 68–69
    pre-competition,
        54–55, 58–60
    pre-exercise, 53–54, 55
    recovery nutrition tips, 73
    rest days, 75–76, 77–80
Nutrigenomics, 51
Nutrition planning. *See*
        also Diet
    age considerations, 91–92
    body composition and
        weight considerations, 92
    children, 100–103
    chronic health issues,
        126–129

Nutrition planning. (*Continued*)
  endurance and
    ultra-endurance
    sports, 107–109
  environmental
    considerations, 93
  high-intensity,
    short-duration
    sports, 112–114
  immune function, 124–126
  men, 95
  overview, 89–90
  recovery, 73, 121–124
  sex considerations, 91
  strength and power
    sports, 109–111
  student athletes, 103–105
  team sports, 111–112
  weight gain, 117–118
  weight loss, 116–117
  weight maintenance,
    118–119
  women, 96–99
Nuts
  Apricot-Coconut
    Granola, 136
  Baked Blueberry
    Oatmeal, 137
  Bueno Breakfast Burrito, 152
  Carrot Cake Muffins, 139
  Cinnamon Quinoa Bowl, 140
  Perfect Pumpkin Energy
    Balls, 147
  Pineapple Fried Rice, 158

O

Oats
  Apricot-Coconut
    Granola, 136
  Baked Blueberry
    Oatmeal, 137
  No-Bake Chocolate Peanut
    Butter Celebration
    Treats, 161
  Peanut Butter Protein
    Balls, 144

Perfect Pumpkin Energy
    Balls, 147
  Sweet Potato Protein
    Pancakes, 142
Omega-3 fatty acids, 24
Omega-6 fatty acids, 24
Osmolality, 6, 9, 82
Overhydration, 7, 9

P

Paleolithic diets, 47
  Almond Butter and Apple
    Sandwiches, 145
  Easy Tender Oven-Baked
    Chicken, 155
  Maple-Dijon–Glazed
    Salmon, 157
Pasta
  Organic Chickpea Fusilli
    with Goat Cheese, 149
Peanut butter
  No-Bake Chocolate Peanut
    Butter Celebration
    Treats, 161
  Peanut Butter Pretzel
    Balls, 146
  Peanut Butter Protein
    Balls, 144
Performance enhancers. *See
  also* Supplements
  performance-enhancing
    drugs (PEDs), 88
  performance supplements,
    86–87
  sports drinks, 62–63,
    75, 82–85
  sports foods, 70–71, 82
Pineapple
  Pineapple Fried Rice, 158
Polyphenols, 87–88
Polysaccharides, 15
Polyunsaturated fats, 22–23, 24
Post-workout recipes
  Almond Butter and Apple
    Sandwiches, 145
  Berry-Cherry Smoothie, 148

Bueno Breakfast Burrito, 152
  Crust-Free Spinach,
    Mushroom, and Cheese
    Quiche, 150
  Organic Chickpea Fusilli
    with Goat Cheese, 149
  Peanut Butter Pretzel
    Balls, 146
  Peanut Butter Protein
    Balls, 144
  Perfect Pumpkin Energy
    Balls, 147
  Slow Cooker Sweet Potato
    Quinoa Curry, 151
Potassium, 4–5, 26
Prebiotics, 48
Pre-competition recipes
  Apricot-Coconut
    Granola, 136
  Baked Blueberry
    Oatmeal, 137
  Blueberry-Stuffed Challah
    French Toast, 138
  Carrot Cake Muffins, 139
  Cinnamon Quinoa
    Bowl, 140
  Over-Easy Grits Bowl, 141
  Sweet Potato Protein
    Pancakes, 142
Pregnancy, 97–98
Pretzels
  Peanut Butter Pretzel
    Balls, 146
Pre-workout recipes
  Apricot-Coconut
    Granola, 136
  Baked Blueberry Oatmeal, 137
  Blueberry-Stuffed Challah
    French Toast, 138
  Carrot Cake Muffins, 139
  Cinnamon Quinoa Bowl, 140
  Over-Easy Grits Bowl, 141
  Sweet Potato Protein
    Pancakes, 142
Probiotics, 86
Processed foods, 38

Protein digestibility-corrected amino acid score (PDCAAS), 21

Proteins
determining quality of, 21
foundation diet planning, 40
overview, 2, 12, 18–19
recommendations, 20
sources of, 19–20

Pumpkin purée
Perfect Pumpkin Energy Balls, 147

Q

Quinoa
Cinnamon Quinoa Bowl, 140
Slow Cooker Sweet Potato Quinoa Curry, 151

R

Recovery, 73, 121–124. See also Rest days

Relative energy deficiency in sport (RED-S), 96

Rest days. See also Rest days recipes
fluid recommendations, 75–76
food recommendations, 77–80
overview, 74

Rest days recipes
Easy Tender Oven-Baked Chicken, 155
Garlic Tahini Dressing, 154
Lazy Beef Bowl, 156
Maple-Dijon–Glazed Salmon, 157
No-Bake Chocolate Peanut Butter Celebration Treats, 161
Pineapple Fried Rice, 158
Sesame-Honey Tempeh with Wild Rice, 159
Southwestern Salad, 160

Resting metabolic rate (RMR), 91

Rice
Pineapple Fried Rice, 158
Sesame-Honey Tempeh with Wild Rice, 159

Rowing, 110–111

Running, 108, 114

S

Salmon
Maple-Dijon–Glazed Salmon, 157

Saturated fats, 21–22

Sex considerations, 91

Sleep deprivation, 104

Snacks. See also
Post-workout recipes;
Pre-competition recipes;
Pre-workout recipes
post-competition, 72
post-workout, 69
pre-competition, 59–60
pre-workout, 58
rest days, 78–79, 80

Soccer, 111

Sodas, 76

Sodium, 4–5, 26, 54, 76

Spinach
Crust-Free Spinach, Mushroom, and Cheese Quiche, 150
Organic Chickpea Fusilli with Goat Cheese, 149
Southwestern Salad, 160

Sports drinks, 62–63, 75, 82–85

Sports foods, 70–71, 82

Starch, 15

Steroids, 88

Strength and power sports, 109–111

Student athletes, 103–105

Sucrose, 14

Sugars, 14

Sunstroke, 11

Supplements
medical, 86
overview, 81
performance, 86–87
polyphenols, 87–88
protein, 19–20
vitamin and mineral, 27–28

Sweat
estimating rate, 65
and fluid loss, 7–8, 54–55

Sweet potatoes
Slow Cooker Sweet Potato Quinoa Curry, 151
Sweet Potato Protein Pancakes, 142

Swimming, 109, 113

T

Tea, 32–33

Team sports, 111–112

Tempeh
Sesame-Honey Tempeh with Wild Rice, 159

Testosterone, 91

Tofu
Bueno Breakfast Burrito, 152

Tomatoes
Organic Chickpea Fusilli with Goat Cheese, 149
Slow Cooker Sweet Potato Quinoa Curry, 151

Training. See also
Post-workout recipes;
Pre-workout recipes
fluids during, 62–63
foods during, 66–67
post-workout fluids, 64
post-workout foods, 68–69
pre-workout fluids, 53–54
pre-workout foods, 56–58
rest days fluids, 75–76
rest days foods, 77–79

Trans fats, 23

U

Ultra-endurance sports, 107–109
Unsaturated fats, 22–23
Urine, 7, 54, 76
U.S. Department of Agriculture (USDA), 38–39

V

Vegan diets, 45–46
   Baked Blueberry Oatmeal, 137
   Bueno Breakfast Burrito, 152
   Perfect Pumpkin Energy Balls, 147
   Slow Cooker Sweet Potato Quinoa Curry, 151
Vegetables, 40, 75
Vegetarian diets, 44–45
   Almond Butter and Apple Sandwiches, 145
   Apricot-Coconut Granola, 136
   Berry-Cherry Smoothie, 148
   Blueberry-Stuffed Challah French Toast, 138
   Carrot Cake Muffins, 139
   Cinnamon Quinoa Bowl, 140
   Crust-Free Spinach, Mushroom, and Cheese Quiche, 150
   Garlic Tahini Dressing, 154
   No-Bake Chocolate Peanut Butter Celebration Treats, 161
   Organic Chickpea Fusilli with Goat Cheese, 149
   Over-Easy Grits Bowl, 141
   Peanut Butter Pretzel Balls, 146
   Peanut Butter Protein Balls, 144
   Pineapple Fried Rice, 158
   Sesame-Honey Tempeh with Wild Rice, 159
   Southwestern Salad, 160
   Sweet Potato Protein Pancakes, 142
Visceral fat, 92
Visualization, 133
Vitamins, 2, 23–28, 86

W

Water, 2, 4–6, 30–32, 75. *See also* Fluid(s)
Water bottles, 33
Weight
   and children, 102
   gain, 117–118
   loss, 116–117
   maintenance, 118–119
   and nutrition planning, 92
Whey, 19–20
Whole grains, 41
Women, 91, 94, 96–99

Y

Yogurt
   Berry-Cherry Smoothie, 148

RECIPE INDEX

A

Almond Butter and Apple
    Sandwiches, 145
Apricot-Coconut Granola, 136

B

Baked Blueberry Oatmeal, 137
Berry-Cherry Smoothie, 148
Blueberry-Stuffed Challah
    French Toast, 138
Bueno Breakfast Burrito, 152

C

Carrot Cake Muffins, 139
Cinnamon Quinoa
    Bowl, 140
Crust-Free Spinach,
    Mushroom, and Cheese
    Quiche, 150

E

Easy Tender Oven-Baked
    Chicken, 155

G

Garlic Tahini
    Dressing, 154

L

Lazy Beef Bowl, 156

M

Maple-Dijon–Glazed
    Salmon, 157

N

No-Bake Chocolate Peanut
    Butter Celebration
    Treats, 161

O

Organic Chickpea Fusilli with
    Goat Cheese, 149
Over-Easy Grits Bowl, 141

P

Peanut Butter Pretzel Balls, 146
Peanut Butter Protein Balls, 144
Perfect Pumpkin Energy
    Balls, 147
Pineapple Fried Rice, 158

S

Sesame-Honey Tempeh with
    Wild Rice, 159
Slow Cooker Sweet Potato
    Quinoa Curry, 151
Southwestern Salad, 160
Sweet Potato Protein
    Pancakes, 142

ACKNOWLEDGMENTS

Writing this book was more rewarding than I could have ever imagined. None of this would have been possible without a few very special people in my life. First off, a genuine thank you to the Callisto Media team, especially Elizabeth Castoria and Vanessa Ta, for believing in me as the author of this book. Second, without the encouragement of my life teammate, Karel, this book would not exist. Over the past 12 years, you have supported my big dreams and crazy ideas. I'm incredibly grateful for all you do, especially the sacrifices you make on my behalf. To my brother, Aaron, and Grandpa Joe, thanks for your support. Mom, I love you. After losing Dad to cancer in 2014, I can't help but be inspired by your strength and renewed zest for life. To my mentors, Judy Molnar, Dr. Gloria Petruzzelli, and Dr. Sharon Brown—you've never stopped believing in me. I appreciate your time, support, and honesty, and thank you for opening doors of opportunity. Joey Mock, without your help, the recipe section of this book would not exist. As a dietitian yourself, you have showcased your attention to detail, patience, and love for cooking with every recipe. To the countless athletes that I've had the pleasure to coach, guide, educate, and inspire over the years, I want to thank you for the everyday learning opportunities and lessons, your trust in me, and the great discussions, questions, and challenges, all of which has kept me on a continuous path of education and professional growth. Last, I'd like to thank my body and mind for staying healthy and resilient throughout this arduous book-writing process and for letting me live such an active life while pursuing my athletic goals.

ABOUT THE AUTHOR

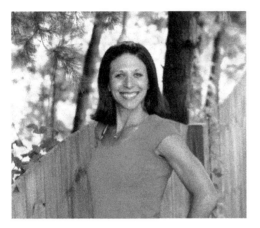

Marni Sumbal, MS, RD, CSSD, LD/N, is a nationally recognized sports dietitian and triathlon coach. Through her renowned, successful private practice, Trimarni Coaching and Nutrition, she helps athletes from around the globe prepare physically and nutritionally for athletic events. She holds a Master of Science degree in exercise physiology and is a board-certified sports dietitian, specializing in endurance sports. Marni is an elite endurance triathlete who has completed 14 Ironman-distance triathlons (including qualifying six times for the Ironman World Championship in Kona, Hawaii) and has successfully finished countless other long-distance triathlon, swimming, running, and cycling events. Getting faster and stronger with age, she won overall amateur female at 2017 Ironman Chattanooga. Marni uses her real-life experiences and formal education to help educate and guide athletes to achieve athletic and nutritional excellence in training and on event day. Her unique "health first, performance second" approach of applying sports and daily nutrition science to real-world settings has gained popularity with many age-group and professional athletes who want practical and realistic nutrition and training strategies when preparing for athletic events. Marni frequently writes for *Triathlete* magazine and has been featured on Ironman.com and TeamUSA.org, and in *Women's Running*, the *New York Times, Runner's World, Women's Health, Women's Running, Bicycling*, and *Men's Journal.* As a public speaker, she was also a regular guest on News4Jax in Jacksonville, Florida, for live TV segments on nutrition. Marni lives near the mountains in Greenville, South Carolina, with her husband, Karel, and three four-legged kids: Campy, Madison, and Smudla. You can contact Marni through her website, www.trimarnicoach.com.

CPSIA information can be obtained
at www.ICGtesting.com
Printed in the USA
BVHW051153111020
590620BV00002B/9